What They're Saying About VITAMINS & YOU

"VITAMINS & YOU is an excellent guidebook
. . . packed with essential information."

Dr. Robert C. Atkins, MD
Author of DR. ATKIN'S
NUTRITION BREAKTHROUGH

"VITAMINS & YOU is an important book—useful, helpful, and innovative."

Joe and Terry Graedon
Authors of THE PEOPLE'S
PHARMACY

"RECOMMENDED."

Dr. Tom Ferguson, MD
Editor: MEDICAL SELF-CARE,
WHOLE EARTH CATALOGUE/
Co EVOLUTION QUARTERLY

"VITAMINS & YOU is a powerful statement about
our deplorable diet . . . a gem of organization and
concise information."

Jane Heimlich
THE CINCINNATI POST

"VITAMINS & YOU is an invaluable guide. It's all there—everything you need to know about vitamins."

"A very valuable addition to the rapidly developing vitamin literature."

"A well-written, comprehensive, practical approach to vitamins by a renowned biochemist-nutritionist. A MUST BOOK."

"A provocative and stimulating book—must reading for the physician and layman alike."

Vitamins & You

ROBERT J. BENOWICZ

BERKLEY BOOKS, NEW YORK

For Katie, Diana, and Duuub

This Berkley book contains the revised
text of the original edition.
It has been completely reset in a type face
designed for easy reading, and was printed
from new film.

VITAMINS & YOU

A Berkley Book / published by arrangement with
Grosset & Dunlap, Inc.

PRINTING HISTORY
Grosset & Dunlap edition published 1979
Revised Berkley edition / October 1981

ISBN: 0-425-05074-2

A BERKLEY BOOK ® TM 757,375
Berkley Books are published by Berkley Publishing Corporation,
200 Madison Avenue, New York, New York 10016.
PRINTED IN THE UNITED STATES OF AMERICA

Contents

1980s Update

Introduction

Why a book about vitamins? Why, indeed, when such a book could save, improve, or prolong your life? Because dietary recklessness has become a national habit that claims, impairs, and shortens tens of millions of lives, concern for improving the American way of eating while achieving and maintaining ideal vitamin intake must become a primary goal for all of us. Proper nutrition—particularly proper vitamin nutrition—can lessen, defer, or prevent the debilitation of aging, promote immunity to infectious disease, improve our general level of health, and help correct the harm done to our bodies by pollution, processed "junk" foods, drugs, and such personal poisons as alcohol and tobacco.

Although our high school textbooks graphically portray some of the crippling vitamin depletion diseases of the recent American past and of the Third World today—rickets, scurvy, beri beri, and pellagra—none of us suffers from those tragic disorders. The dramatic injury and impairment of such exotic hygiene class "horribles" are as much relics of our nation's history as silent movies, gramophones, and the five-cent cigar. They have been replaced by species of slow and subtle killers, the chronic degenerative diseases that take root in the soil of personal malnutrition—particularly vitamin malnutrition—and flower among us with all of the haunting familiarity of double-digit inflation, decaying cities, and the neutron bomb.

Heart and circulatory disorders, the many varieties of cancer, and diabetes now constitute the principal causes of mortality in our modern industrial age. Nonlethal arthritis and rheumatism are similarly prevalent and share many common characteristics with their deadly counterparts. Most of these dread disorders and their insidious cousins (many forms of schizophrenia, autism, and other mental illnesses) seem to be *metabolic* diseases that result from conflicts between our inherited biochemistry and the environmental conditions in which it must function. Although there is little we can personally do to alter the quality of the air we breathe or the water we drink, there _are_ significant steps we can take to maximize our chances for improved and prolonged good health through careful attention to the foods we eat and the vitamins we consume.

Because of government's failure to cope with the social, economic, and physical ills that plague our age, it is difficult to keep faith with bureaucracies that have shown continual disdain for our nutritional fitness and wellbeing. When federal agencies assure us that our daily metabolic need for vitamins can be met with a spoon and an everyday bowl of quite ordinary and wholly unremarkable breakfast cereal, it is wise to remember that those same custodians of national health have conducted our "War on Cancer" by ignoring the fact that more than 40 percent of all malignancy has its origins in nutritional causes. For years they have poured more than 98 percent of our research dollars into areas of inquiry that have failed to prevent or cure this awful disease, and it is taking the action of an outraged Congress to reorder priorities. Since it is already known that vitamin C prevents the

breakdown of fertilizer nitrates and food-additive nitrites
into carcinogenic nitrosamines, it is well within the realm
of possibility that the stimulus needed to convert ordinary
cells into cancerous aberrants may come from prolonged
—albeit marginal—vitamin starvation. Indeed, we may
wonder about the hostility of our governmental and medical authorities toward the *testing* of ascorbic acid—or
vitamin C—for the prevention and/or cure of cancer. Although the substance has been found effective by highly
respected national health agencies and cancer-care specialists in foreign countries, until very recently our medical and research establishment steadfastly refused to test
and measure the effectiveness of Vitamin C. When our
health-care custodians dismiss the potential value of
promising preventives or cures for cancer *before they have
been subjected to objective scientific evaluation,* it is later
than any of us thinks.

Although nutritional misadventure is the leading
cause of death in America today, official documents do not
describe fatality in terms of knives and forks, preferring
more conventional verdicts that include the various forms
of heart and circulatory disorders, cancer, and the complications arising from diabetes. Eight out of every ten of
us now die from one of these diseases, few of which have
an infectious origin. Most are chronic, degenerative disorders that take many years, if not decades, to develop.
Although the once-dread viral and bacterial killers have
succumbed to the skilled techniques and practices of modern medicine, our elaborate and costly health-care system
is a lumbering dinosaur slow to respond to recent and
dramatic alteration in disease patterns that now substitute
debilitation for contagion. Its awesome hardware, powerful drugs, and sophisticated scalpels are virtually worth-
less for the prevention, and only marginally effective for
the treatment, of the now prominent diseases that enervate
and destroy us.

Failure to recognize and respond to the profound
differences in the nature, origin, and development of degenerative disorders and infectious illness is a serious

charge that must be laid at the door of our national health-care custodians. The chronic and killing diseases that plague us are the probable products of the body's ultimate collapse in the face of the profound shocks and prolonged abuses it must sustain in its contemporary struggle for survival. The air we breathe, the water we drink, and—above all—the food we eat are inextricably linked to the subtle and pernicious deterioration of bone, fiber, and sinew. Because life is a continual compromise between an organism's ideal metabolic requirements and the actual quality of the fuels, fluids, and gases that support it, any inferior, alien, or toxic input is apt to undermine health and well-being. The fact of air and water pollution is well known. That the quality of our foods has undergone a similar sullying and suborning—particularly during the past two decades—is less generally recognized. With our uncritical substitution of industrially manipulated, processed products in the place of whole, fresh, and natural foods, we have invited nutritional subversives into our kitchens and dining rooms. Although calorically rich, our chemicalized cuisine is vitamin poor. That there is a significant correlation between the increased incidence of chronic disease and the decline in quality of our foods is more than mere coincidence.

Since every cell in our body requires vitamins to carry on the business of life, a life without these essential compounds is soon no life at all. Because of its extraordinary biochemical resilience, our metabolism can maintain itself —albeit at minimal levels of effectiveness—so long as small quantities of all the different vitamins are supplied to it. If cells or tissues are deprived of these nutrients for any length of time, permanent injury or death is sure to follow. Admitting no more than the danger of total depletion or exhaustion, the Food and Drug Administration (FDA) instructs us to consume Recommended Daily Allowances (U.S. RDAs) of all the various vitamins. The quantities it suggests are held *adequate* to prevent the devastating deficiency disorders, such as scurvy, among most healthy Americans. That these mandated amounts—

obtainable in a daily serving of a few "enriched" breakfast gruels—achieve their stated purpose is reasonably certain. That they can supply us with the *ideal* quantities our metabolism requires for *optimum* function is questionable. Impressive evidence suggests that vitamin concentrations sufficient to prevent clinical deficiency diseases but lower than those needed for the most efficient biochemical function keep large numbers of us in a state of physical limbo—suspended between the poles of outright sickness and genuine good health. Prolonged existence at marginal levels of metabolic effectiveness takes its inevitable toll by undermining vital cells and tissues, thereby making the body vulnerable to chronic degenerative disorders and acute infectious diseases. With its advocacy of vitamin intake designed to stave off clinical deficiency rather than to achieve maximum biochemical function, the FDA encourages national malnutrition as it promotes vitamin starvation.

Support for rationing of vitamins comes from a pair of unlikely bedfellows—our medical cartels and corporate giants of the food industry. Agribusiness interests benefit from minimal U.S. RDAs because their products appear nutritionally richer at lower levels of recommended intake. The purposes of American Medical Association (AMA) opposition to vitamin supplementation are less certain. It has been suggested that we would all be taking vitamins at a physician's behest if the FDA had succeeded in its recent attempts to classify supplement products with more than 150 percent of any U.S. RDA as prescription drugs.[1] Such allegations of venality may be viewed with some skepticism since standard medical practice recognizes many legitimate uses for supplementation. The stated concern of most medical spokesmen—that the personal and unregulated enthusiasm for vitamins may lead to their abuse—is plausible. So is the reflex tendency of party-line physicians to suggest that the proponents of greater vitamin intake are all charlatans, hucksters, and

---

1. Congress and the President struck down this effort as an infringement upon an individual's freedom of nutritional choice.

quacks. Their medical training and that of most American doctors ignores the role of nutrition—let alone vitamins—in both health and disease. The orthodox medical practitioner is apt to know no more than the layman about how the food he eats becomes an integral part of his body tissue, and his disdain for supplementation belongs to the realm of political opinion rather than sound scientific judgement. However, increasing numbers of physicians—frustrated by the impotence of their surgical knives and prescription pads—encourage the use of relatively large quantities of vitamins *to promote maximum health and prevent premature body deterioration and eventual disease.* Whether or not you or your family are advised to supplement your diets will probably depend on the doctor you choose rather than any authoritarian edict issued from a medical-association boardroom.

Because professional journals and the daily press bear frequent and poignant witness to the often tragic results of postponing proper medical care in favor of some nutritional fad or fancy, it is not surprising that health-care officials and the medical establishment share concerns about any public inclination to use vitamins and other dietary supplements as if they were drugs. That they express such concerns is admirable. That they resolutely deny the potential benefits of proper nutritional supplementation and attempt to suppress the sale, distribution, and use of vitamin products because beasts of the "common herd" are nutritional buffoons is an outrage.

The history of science and medicine is littered with the corpses of academic and bureaucratic experts who rejected novel and valid ideas that contradicted their narrow notions of scientific truth. It has often been laymen—unencumbered by hoary preconceptions and excess intellectual baggage—who have first realized the value of new and original thinking. In America today, the use of supplementary vitamins is no longer limited to health food freaks, faddists, and the great unwashed. We are far from being the village idiots governmental health-care agencies and the orthodox medical establishment believe us to be.

Our nationwide preoccupation with physical fitness, passion for jogging, pursuit of nutritionally whole foods, and concern about pollution reflect a gut understanding that the prevalent diseases of modern times have their origin in a lifetime of injurious living and eating habits in an increasingly toxic environment. Concern for ensuring good health *while still healthy* reveals an intuitive knowledge that failure of the human body doesn't happen magically or at any particular, fixed, or given moment. It reveals our passionate desire to prevent the degenerative, crippling, and humiliating illnesses that—with growing frequency—undermine the young, condemn the mature, and make the aged body a prison. People increasingly reject medical practice that is powerless to intervene on their behalf until a dread and debilitating disease has taken hold of them. Popular impulse demands individualized, preventive protection from the corrosive effects of harmful personal habits and the biological encroachment of an alien and hostile environment.

Because we obviously are and continue to become what we eat, the quality of our foodstuffs is a natural target for scrutiny among those Americans concerned about their present and future health. There is growing public awareness that current agricultural practices and ingenious methods for processing, packaging, and preserving our foods rob them of intrinsic nutritional worth. Vitamins suffer most severely from such technological manipulations, and our penchant for repeated cooking and reheating of modern convenience foods adds physical insult to their biochemical injury. To supplement a daily diet in compensation for such nutritional impoverishment is logical and desirable. It may well be necessary for maintaining our good health.

Although it is true that far too many have been susceptible to Madison Avenue's regular conversion of dietary dross into nutritional gold by proclaiming the vitamin virtues of its much-touted products, we do not have to succumb to such promotional hype or remain the passive victims of health-establishment indifference. While personal health and nutrition are inextricably linked factors in a complex equation involving many as yet unknown or poorly understood variables, the fact that vitamins have a critical function in that relationship is undeniable. Although there is much to be learned and the last word on the subject of nutrition has yet to be written, we can take individual steps to optimally fulfill our vitamin needs and be certain to increase our chances for good health and well-being. The effort isn't always easy. It is worth the try.

VITAMINS & YOU

Your Diet: Overfed and Undernourished?

Tell me what you eat, and I'll tell you what you are.
— BRILLAT-SAVARIN

If you are typical of most Americans, you have little difficulty getting enough calories to fuel your metabolic furnace. With more than half the adult population measurably overweight, it is easy to point with pride to the agricultural enlightenment of a nation whose principal nutritional problems involve an overabundance rather than a scarcity of foodstuffs. Yet it is the quality, not the quantity, of metabolic input that ultimately ensures or undermines your health.

Because your body is so nearly perfect a machine, it can function for years—even when negligently fueled—without a serious breakdown or perceptible complaint. This capacity for compromise between its ideal metabolic requirements and the actual raw materials you place at its disposal is a mixed blessing. Although the body's inherent flexibility protects you at times of chemical adversity or deficiency, its adaptability is finite and the price of repeated assault is ultimately paid in the coin of ill health or outright disease.

To understand that the air, water, and food you consume must affect your body's exquisite and complex functioning is easy. To perceive the insidious effects of exposure to inferior, sullied, or adulterated forms of these metabolic raw ingredients is difficult, if not impossible. Just as surely as you will be unable to sense any loss of body function with the fumes from a single cigarette, the cumulative effects of smoking will eventually impair your health and shorten your life. In a similar fashion the rapid befouling of America's air and water resources is predictably playing imperceptible but inexorable havoc with the metabolism of every man, woman, and child. The quantity, quality, and variety of pollutants is staggering. They cast a thick and noxious pall that stretches from coast to coast. They permeate once-pristine watersheds and create aquatic deserts where no life can survive. To predict the effects of such environmental pollution is difficult. Not until long after the Industrial Revolution had shrouded the English midlands in a darkening gloom did anyone realize that dimming the sun inhibited the skin's normal formation of vitamin D and produced thousands of bewildered cripples.

To escape contact with twentieth-century pollutants is impossible. Coping with their disruption of normal biochemical processes is a function of your unique metabolism. While response will vary from individual to individual, no scientist can be easy about the overall adaptability of the human race. As the by-products of highly artificial technological processes, most pollutant molecules have never before been part of the environment. As a species, man lacks the protection usually provided by millions of years of adaptive coexistence with potential poisons. The implications are ominous.

That American food is subtly undermined in a fashion similar to the suborning of national air and water resources is a reality. Subversion begins with the animal and plant sources of our food supply. As living organisms with unique metabolic needs, crop plants and livestock are as vulnerable to the general decline in environmental quality as you are. With the introduction of farming methods that value profit over nutrition, of food-processing techniques that sacrifice quality for expediency, and of advertising practices that make virtues of vices, decline in the effectiveness of your food is inevitable. Famine amidst plenty is a real possibility. Malnutrition is undeniably on the rise. You may well be one of the overfed and undernourished.

WHAT HAVE THEY DONE TO OUR FOOD?

The eating habits of a nation can change rapidly. Economic pressures, historical events, new agricultural practices, climatic vagaries, population explosions, media advertising, alteration in lifestyles, and the refinements of food technologies have all had a hand in profoundly changing the American diet during the twentieth century. Through the sophisticated use of manufactured fertilizers, pesticides, insecticides, growth hormones, and a knowledge of selective breeding, American farmers achieve an unprecedented yield of foodstuffs per acre of arable land. Newer methods for harvest, transport, storage, and preservation make possible an unparalleled range of food choices the year round. Advances in food chemistry continue to produce a bewildering number of novel ways to combine basic food elements to tease the palate and tempt the pocketbook.

If a turn-of-the-century American could be resurrected and propelled into the modern supermarket, he would be staggered by the vast range of available products —18,000 instead of the 100 or so of his General Store; by the dazzling packaging that seals food into transparent plastics, metallic papers, and vacuum tins; and by the refrigerators, crispers, and freezers designed for both the preservation and display of this bounty. He might well conclude that his children's children had re-entered the Garden of Eden. You may be less sanguine.

Although the life of your turn-of-the-century grandfather or great grandfather was darkened by the specter of death from infectious diseases, his life expectancy at 40 was but 4.5 years less than your own. Persuasive arguments are made that the benefits of eliminating death by infection are largely offset by deterioration in the integrity of basic foodstuffs. The process began more than a century ago and had its origin in economic expediency, misplaced aesthetics, and biochemical ignorance. It reflects a decline persuasively linked to a spectacular increase in the incidence of such degenerative ills as heart disease, arthritis, diabetes, and cancer.

Staple Foods: The Impoverished Basics

Because it is easy to confuse lavish quantities and seductive qualities of available food products with nutritional riches, it is equally easy to assume that the American diet of today is superior to that of the past. In fact, most of our highly elaborated and fabricated foods are compounded from a modest number of basic ingredients, similar in kind but inferior in quality to those relied upon by our forebears.

SUGAR: A SWEET SUBVERSIVE

During the nineteenth century Americans sweetened their cakes, breads, pies, and other pastries with molasses, natural honey, maple syrup, and unrefined sugar. Because each of these substances concentrates the nutritional output of its plant or animal parent, each is intrinsically rich in the very carbohydrates, minerals, and vitamins that attract bacteria and subject it to spoilage. As the nation's population crowded into cities during the last quarter of the nineteenth century, farmers faced the enormous problem of delivering such perishable but prized foodstuffs to increasingly distant markets. Refined sugar—extracted from the raw sap of beet roots or cane with high heat, charcoal filters, and acid washes—provided an expedient substitute. The "refined" product, table sugar, had to be 99.5 percent pure sucrose by law. It contained none of its original vitamins and only a trace of its original minerals.

In its white crystalline form, sucrose won instant approval at Victorian tea tables. Its immunity to spoilage[1] appealed to farmers and food processors. Its sweetening powers proved seductive and enduring.

Sucrose addiction has steadily increased through the century so that today the *per capita* intake of refined sugar is more than 100 pounds per person per year and accounts for more than one quarter of the daily calories consumed by "average" Americans. Most of this enormous quantity is masked as an additive, not only to pastry, jam, and candy, but as a subtle though primary ingredient of breads, cereals, processed fruits and vegetables, soft drinks, and even meats.

The wholesale introduction of sucrose into the American diet has had enormous impact on the nation's health. An appalling increase in tooth decay—particularly among children—was the most immediate and obvious result. The early appearance of dental cavities has become a routine expectation of childhood, and its elimination is unlikely as food processors continue to develop, produce, and promote sucrose-rich cupcakes, candies, colas, and cereals aimed at the highly susceptible and vulnerable youth market. Adding fluorine to water and training more dentists has been a curious response to a major health problem.

A more insidious effect of sucrose consumption is its long-term assault on your metabolism. In substituting refined sugar for the natural varieties found in honey, maple sugar, and molasses, a tremendous burden is placed on the body's capacity to produce or absorb insulin, the pancreatic hormone that regulates levels of sugar in the bloodstream. Any introduction of sucrose into the body triggers release of the hormone.

Inability to produce insulin may result from an inherited defect which manifests itself early in childhood. This genetic disorder is rare and was probably the only form of

---

1. Robbed of their vitamin and mineral riches, sugar and other processed staples lose their nutritional completeness and fail to attract the microbial and insect pests drawn to nutritionally whole and unrefined products.

diabetes known in the nineteenth century. Today, diabetes and its side effects rank third after circulatory diseases and cancer as the leading cause of death among Americans. Estimates place its incidence as high as 60 percent among those over 55 and as high as 80 percent among those who live beyond 70. In contrast with inherited childhood forms, adult, or late-onset, diabetes is an acquired disease. Its startling incidence in the twentieth century corresponds to the widespread use of refined sugar. The biochemical explanation is straightforward. By ingesting large amounts of sucrose throughout a lifetime, you place cells of the pancreas under constant and abnormal stress, leading either to the exhaustion of their ability to synthesize insulin or to the loss of the capacity of tissue cells to absorb the hormone from the bloodstream. Diabetes is the result.

As the dangers of sucrose have been recognized—more for the waistline than the metabolism—alarming numbers of Americans have acquired the habit of foregoing their sugar without loss of their sweet. Sodium saccharin, a coal-tar derivative and sugar substitute, is entering the American diet with a rapidity reminiscent of the turn-of-the-century intrusion of sucrose. Although intended for use by diabetics, who must eliminate or control their intake of sugar, saccharin and its chemical relatives are becoming the sweetening staple for many in a youth-oriented, weight-conscious society. Artificially "sugared" candy, soft drinks, ice cream, bread, and pastries are now as American as apple pie. That compounds such as saccharin or the cyclamates satisfy a craving for sweet without delivering the calories of sucrose is undeniable. That the long-term effects of consuming such agents are trivial is highly debatable. On evidence that they produce malignancy in laboratory animals, the Food and Drug Administration (FDA) has banned the inclusion of cyclamates in all foods. Acting on similar evidence, the FDA now requires that all foods containing saccharin bear the warning that "this product contains saccharin which has been determined to cause cancer in laboratory animals." Whether this caution will be any more effective than that included on cigarette labels remains to be seen. Whether you can have your sweet and safely eat it too is the question. There can be little doubt that the replacement of such natural agents as molasses, honey, and maple sugar with refined sugars or saccharin is a blow to your nutritional well-being.

FLOUR: THEY SAVE THE CHAFF

Much of the history of western civilization can be written in terms of the success or failure of its wheat crop. Good health, social welfare, and economic prosperity are the traditional hallmarks of bumper harvests, while famine, migration, warfare, and/or impoverishment are typical hardships of failed plantings. Russia's current need to purchase American wheat is but a single incident in the ongoing saga of human dependence on this precious commodity. Its nutritional gold lies in the kernel or fruit, which contains a rich and concentrated store of protein, carbohydrate, unsaturated fats, vitamins, and minerals. By drying and grinding, wheat kernels are converted to flour, the familiar and ubiquitous staple of breads, cakes, pasta, and pastry.

Until the end of the nineteenth century, the milling or grinding of wheat into flour was a rather crude affair. It involved the use of massive stone wheels that reduced the kernels to a coarse meal. Because the product was so nutritionally rich, it was a highly perishable commodity, subject to microbial contamination, insect infestation, and rodent attack. Its rough texture yielded breads and cakes of a similar nature. Economic expediency and the aesthetic tastes of the age demanded a less vulnerable, more refined substitute. The demand was met by crushing the raw wheat between immense pressure rollers, which reduced the kernels to a fine dust. Sifting out the cruder and discolored portions with filters and bleaching the end product to hygienic whiteness using strong acids or other oxidants produced a final, refined flour remarkably resistant to decay. It yielded desirably light pastries, which met the aesthetic demands of the most fastidious eye.

Unfortunately, the refinement process—then and now—removes many of the essential food elements that make stone-milled flour so nutritionally viable. Along with the unsightly germ, bran, and husk go most of the protein, all of the unsaturated oils, and most of the vitamins and minerals. It is little wonder that refined and bleached flour is so immune to attack and contamination.

The universal military draft and World War II brought standardized medical checkups for millions of American men. That significant numbers were found unfit for service because of gross nutritional deficiencies led to an intensive investigation of the national diet. Refined and bleached flour, the principal ingredient in many foods, was found seriously wanting. The FDA, recognizing that processing techniques were robbing foods of essential nutritional elements, ordered that flour and other basic foods be "enriched" with minimum amounts of thiamin (vitamin B_1), riboflavin (vitamin B_2), niacin (vitamin B_3), and the minerals calcium and iron. At the time of this enrichment order, the commissioner of the FDA noted that adequate nutrition was more certainly assured through the use of unprocessed foods, e.g. stone-ground flour, than through reliance on vitamin-fortified processed foods, e.g. refined flour. Although simply complying with FDA requirements, food processors cynically confounded the public by declaring a nutritional dividend with their "enriched" product—even though they were forced, rather than volunteered, to restore some of the essential food elements lost in processing. Others, equally devious, implied that their enrichment procedures supplied any and all missing food elements. Nothing could have been further from the truth.

Comparison of the nutritional information panel of a typical enriched, bleached, and refined flour with that of a common wheat germ product reveals the nutritional bankruptcy of the processors' claims. One ounce of wheat germ typically contains 8 times the amount of protein, 3 times the amount of unsaturated fatty acids, 3 times the amount of thiamin, 1½ times the amount of riboflavin, and equal amounts of iron and calcium as the comparable ounce of flour. Present in the wheat germ, but absent from the refined flour, are significant quantities of vitamins C, D, E, pantothenic acid, pyridoxine (vitamin B_6), folic acid, and such minerals as phosphorus, magnesium, zinc, and copper. Can there be any question that your turn-of-the-century grandfather enjoyed far fuller and richer nutrition with his stone-ground flour than you do today with your highly refined, bleached, and "enriched" substitute?

Wheat is not the only grain to suffer nutritional insult. Similar sins are perpetrated against rice by hulling and polishing. The torturing of cereal grains through flaking, baking, popping, and toasting robs them of essential food elements—particularly vitamins.

VEGETABLE OILS: ADULTERATED FAT

A combination of technological, economic, and medical factors accounts for the dramatic incursion of nutritionally emasculated vegetable oils into the American diet during the past twenty-five years. Although man has pressed nutritionally rich oil from the olive since time out of mind, he has only recently learned to extract similar products from a host of beans, seeds, grains, and nuts. The price of this newly acquired skill is a dietary penance. Whereas the oil of the olive is so concentrated that the soft fruit requires no more than mechanical pressing for extraction, the fruits of the soybean, corn, safflower, and peanut must be subjected to extreme measures before yielding their oils. In some cases pulverizing the fruit, heating it to more than 300°F., and then forcing it through a corkscrew press will produce adequate yields. Such "expeller-pressed" oils are clearly less damaged than those claimed by "solvent extraction" methods. The latter and more common process involves pressure-cooking the pulverized fruit with a petroleum distillate to dissolve the oil. The petroleum solvent is driven off by heating to temperatures approaching 500°F. Residues of the fruit pulp are removed by filtration and the extracted oil is subjected to the indignities of bleaching and deodorizing. The product, a viscous liquid of innocuous taste and color, may be bottled as cooking oil or hydrogenated to form vegetable solids for use in margarine, ice cream, candy, peanut butter, yogurt, and a host of processed "junk" foods.

Although the solvent extraction method destroys most fat-soluble vitamins, essential fatty acids, some protein, and many vitamins of the B complex, it is now the principal means by which contemporary vegetable oils are produced. That such nutritionally assaulted and weakened products have supplanted once-favored meat, butter, and lard as primary sources of essential fats in the American diet may seem baffling. The reasons, if not obvious, are compelling and unfortunate. Economic necessity often overrides nutritional good sense. Animal products are hard on the pocketbook and the substitution of cheaper plant products keeps pennies in the purse. The very innocuousness of vegetable oil is a food chemist's dream as he uses its neutrality to advantage in the elaboration of many "new and different" foods. To his corporate superior, a man with his eye on the balance sheet, the abundance and low cost of vegetable oils make them ideal substitutes for more traditional and expensive ingredients —particularly since the consumer doesn't usually recognize or seem to care about the substitution. Public alarm over the medical establishment's concern with blood level concentrations of cholesterol gives final impetus to the growing preference for vegetable oils. Many consumers now view their use as nickels in the bag of medical and fiscal good health. You may wonder at the wisdom of such economies.

The Nutritional Cannibals:
Calorie Rich and Vitamin Poor

You may legitimately ask how the decline in quality of staple foods affects you and your metabolism. Although processing compromises the nutritional integrity of whole sugar, wheat, rice, cereal grains, and vegetable oils, it clearly does not destroy all food value. If it did, Americans would suffer from starvation rather than obesity.

Because some of the nutrients in raw foods have remarkable molecular stability, they can withstand the chemical and physical assaults of the refinement process. Carbohydrates and minerals are the most resistant to abuse. Although stress causes proteins and fats to disintegrate into their respective amino acid and fatty acid components, this disassembling is an ordinary function of human digestion. Such breakdown outside the body does not compromise the capacity to utilize these essential nutrients in synthesizing your own unique proteins and fats. Among all the nutritional elements, vitamins are the most vulnerable to brutalization. They are easily destroyed by heat, light, air, and chemical processing. Once degraded, their components are of no nutritional value, since your cells are incapable of reassembling them from any raw material.

Although the principal crime of processing staple foods is the decimation of vitamins, all intrinsic food elements with the exception of carbohydrates suffer partial if not total diminution in concentration or function. Refined sugar contains none of the plant protein or vegetable oils of the original cane or beet. Of a wide range of minerals, only traces of copper and iron remain. Elimination of the germ, bran, and husk from wheat removes all of its natural oils, most of its protein, and much of its mineral content. Refined sugar, flour, rice, and cereal grains are virtually pure forms of carbohydrate. Processed vegetable oil is almost exclusively fat.

Because carbohydrates and fats constitute the principal energy sources or fuels for your metabolic machinery, the consumption of refined sugar, flour, and vegetable oil assures you of a rich caloric bank account with which to power your body. You may wonder why a diet rich in refined carbohydrates and fats, complemented by an ample intake of protein, shouldn't meet all your nutritional needs.

Although the ingestion of carbohydrates, proteins, and fats is essential to life, your body cannot make use of these nutrients without vitamins and minerals. The biochemical processes of metabolism—*particularly the utilization of proteins, carbohydrates, and fats*—require enzymes. Various vitamins and minerals play a critical role in the proper functioning of specific enzymes. Since all food elements work synergistically, or cooperatively, less-than-optimal concentrations of any vitamin or mineral limit or impair the effectiveness of your whole metabolism. When in recent years the United Nations rushed protein supplements to African countries where children were suffering from the severe protein deficiency disease known as *kwashiorkor,* consumption of the supplement caused blindness among many of the victims. Evidently, the sudden ingestion of protein placed excessive demands on already enfeebled body stores of the vitamin A necessary to metabolize the nutrient. Exhaustion of the vitamin A reserves produced a characteristic and irreversible loss of vision. In a similar fashion the consumption of calorie-rich and vitamin-poor processed sugar, flour, and vegetable oil exerts a tremendous strain on your tissue stores of essential vitamins. The burden of replenishing adequate concentrations of these nutrients rests with the balance of your diet. That the ubiquitous frozen, canned, and dehydrated convenience foods of today can compensate for the vitamin drain created by the refined staples, which constitute as much as 50 percent of your daily food intake, is highly questionable. Refined sugar, flour, rice, cereal grains, and vegetable oils are nutritionally subversive. They are vitamin cannibals.

AGRIBUSINESS AND OUR CHEMICAL CUISINE

The problems of profitably providing safe, nutritious, and appetizing food for more than 220 million Americans are enormous. Gone are the days when an essentially rural and agrarian people either raised their own foodstuffs or lived in towns and villages wholly supplied with the bounty of local farms. With more than 70 percent of the population now living in massive and sprawling urban centers, the distance from farm to fork and pasture to palate has lengthened tremendously. Direct contact with the land is a memory; the suburban child is more apt to associate the source of his food with the supermarket than with the soil.

As the physical and psychological gulf between you and your food supply widens, the logistics of feeding you and your family become infinitely more complex and demanding. They are no longer the province of the small independent farm and farmer whose responsibility once extended from planting the seed and birthing the calf to delivery of fresh meat, milk, and produce to your doorstep. Responsibility increasingly rests with a handful of monolithic corporations—the agribusiness giants—whose capacities for growing, harvesting, processing, and marketing of foodstuffs are awesome. They have largely organized food production on a nationwide scale. Given the scope of their operations, their system is a marvel of efficiency. Unfortunately, so vast and far-flung an empire introduces a host of interferents into the process of translating food from the garden to your gullet. The orange juice you drank with breakfast this morning may have been plucked from a Florida tree more than three years ago. En route to your table it may have passed through more than forty different stages in processing and handling. Each step took time and offered opportunities for the tampering and adulteration that have subtly converted the American diet into an essentially chemical cuisine.

Down on the Farm: Chemical Warfare

Nature has blessed our country with more than a quarter of the earth's topsoil, long growing seasons, and a temperate climate. Realizing the maximum potential of this bounty is a primary goal of twentieth-century technology. Its successes have been tremendous. They are the envy of the world. Although considerable credit belongs to the farm-implement manufacturers, irrigation engi-

neers, and geneticists, it is the extraordinary resourceful-
ness of the agricultural chemist that accounts for the most
spectacular gains in productivity. His laboratory continues to yield fertilizers that restore and enrich soils in ways
that genuinely improve upon Nature.

Essential minerals are absorbed into the bodies of
crop plants through their roots and are often concentrated
in the ripened fruit. Harvesting effectively removes the
mineral-laden fruit and leaves the mother earth poorer in
her supply of essential elements. The use of such natural
and "organic" fertilizers as manure derived from animals
grazing on the land only partially restores the missing
nutrients. Some of the minerals are incorporated into the
animal's body. If the soil on which the animal grazes is
initially mineral-deficient, his metabolism will be impaired
and his waste materials will reflect the original deficit. By
creating fertilizers that can correct soil deficiencies, agricultural technology provides the means for reclaiming
millions of acres of marginal crop and pasture land while
ensuring the continued richness of currently prime soil.
The importance of this achievement cannot be denied. It
can be overvalued, as it has encouraged other chemical
technologies of less certain utility and merit.

In his zeal for improving upon Nature, the chemist
has created whole classes of compounds whose initial benefits to agricultural productivity seemed immense. During
the past three decades hundreds of the nation's laboratories have produced thousands of entirely new and highly
toxic molecules that were rapidly marketed as pesticides,
insecticides, and fungicides. Scientific caution was scat-
tered to the winds while these new compounds were
rushed into general use. Their effectiveness in eliminating
or controlling the microbial, insect, and rodent pests that
had perennially decimated crops and plagued herds is
awesome. With their widespread application and repeated
use, per-acre yields of plant and animal products skyrock-
eted. Not until they permeated the very pith and marrow
of the environment did scientists recognize the perils of
indiscriminately releasing such impersonal, manmade poisons into Nature. The loss of wildlife, the pollution of

water, and other disruptions of delicate ecological balances are ominous. Of more immediate concern is the effect of these highly toxic compounds on your own metabolism.

Every American has ingested DDT. Although banned from use some years ago, it resides in your liver and will remain with you until death. Like so many related but less familiar agricultural poisons, it is not subject to breakdown by your body chemistry. Among certain birds DDT disrupts the utilization of calcium and leads to the formation of eggs whose shells are too weak to resist the pressure of the brooding hen. Its long-term effects on your metabolism are unknown. The toxic effects of other widely used and commercially available pesticides, such as Dieldrin and Aldrin, are more immediately injurious—even lethal—and were long recognized as such before their use and that of even more potent ones was forbidden. As any mystery fan or pharmacologist knows, the human body can absorb small quantities of such lethal poisons as arsenic or thallium over long periods of time without the appearance of serious or perceptible symptoms. Although tolerance for the toxin may increase, when levels of tissue saturation are reached, death is inevitable. In a similar fashion, thoughtful scientists fear that the gradual accumulation and concentration of agricultural poisons in the human body will impair your health even if they do not prove fatal.

Although the FDA has now banned many of the more insidious pesticides and has severely restricted the use of thousands of others, the complete obliteration of such compounds is now impossible. Repeated exposure has eliminated vulnerable strains of microbe, insect, and rodent, and favored resistant varieties that would decimate crops without chemical controls. Protection of your food supply now depends on these compounds. Whether you can survive their long-term use as they continue to collect in various parts of the body is an unanswered question.

Although no one can legitimately accuse agribusiness of intended evil in its pursuit and development of pesticides and other agricultural poisons, understanding that your good health and nutrition are not its primary concerns can help explain how this double-edged chemical sword got loose in the land. As a commercial enterprise, its principal goal is profit. At the farming end of the operation a premium is placed on plant or animal crops that produce a high yield with rapid and uniform growth. Quick and even maturation, resistance to disease, and hardiness in the face of climatic extremes are prized characteristics. Ultimate weight and appearance, rather than nutritional endowment, are essential concerns. When diethylstilbestrol (DES), a hormone, is fed to calves, they gain weight far more rapidly than animals denied the drug. Although DES has been shown to cause cancer in humans, the major food conglomerates have fought its ban with tooth and claw. When the interests of the consumer and the corporation converge, everyone benefits. When they don't, you know who takes precedence. Don't be fooled by the beguiling advertising of the contented cows and complacent corn with which agribusiness attempts to identify your best interests with its own.

From the Factory: Process or Perish

Before 1940 fewer than 10 percent of the foods on a grocer's shelves had been chemically waylaid in transit between harvest and home. With the development of K-rations during World War II the Federal Government gave unwitting but decisive legitimacy to the fledgling food-processing industry. Its growth in intervening years has been phenomenal. Its effect on the diet and eating habits of Americans has been as catastrophic as it has been incalculable.

Of the more than 18,000 food items available at your supermarket, over 80 percent, or 15,000, have undergone major chemical processing and reprocessing. Milder forms of manipulation include the freezing, drying, and canning of fruits, vegetables, meats, poultry, and fish. Although such techniques do not appreciably alter the caloric value of your food, they do wreak havoc on its vitamin content. More brutal processing involves various methods of chemical and physical refinement, degradation, reconstitution, bleaching, boiling, and deodorizing. Often these represent secondary assaults on food prepared with already adulterated sugar, flour, and vegetable oils. Most convenience foods have undergone this double jeopardy, including such American dietary favorites as breakfast squares, pot pies, commercial "pastries," TV dinners, dried soups, pop tarts, processed cheese, potato chips, crackers, cookies, doughnuts, ice cream, fruit ades, and soft drinks.

THE STAFF OF LIFE IS A BROKEN ROD

Although you may be aware that convenience foods tend to be nutritionally bankrupt, you may not know that some traditionally regarded nutritional "giants" are nearly as impoverished. White bread, once the staff of life, is now a broken rod. Its confabulation from tortured wheat, sugar, and vegetable oil makes it one of the most voracious of vitamin cannibals. Although its "enrichment" is touted as capable of building your body in many ways, only a portion (8 of 23) of its original nutrients are actually restored, and a number of those are immediately lost in the processes that expand a small fistful of dough into the usual football-sized loaf. Whatever "enrichment" remains following inflation and baking is probably consumed in digestion and metabolism of the bread itself.

THE GREAT BREAKFAST CEREAL SWINDLE

More flagrant betrayal of your nutritional trust involves those breakfast cereals that broadly proclaim their virtues in bold face and bury their numerous vices in fine print. After concoction by flaking, baking, puffing, popping, cracking, or otherwise abusing wheat, oats, rice, corn, or other grains, such products contain little besides raw carbohydrate in the form of starch. Large amounts of sugar, salt, and corn syrup must be added to make them moderately palatable. Because the quantity of sweetening is so large, diabetics must forego these metabolic marvels, and those on salt-free or salt-restricted regimens must do so as well. Even in the absence of such dietary prohibitions you may wonder about the promised nutritional riches of your favorite cereal. The scant half-cup of milk you pour over the top contains more than twice the available protein, 5 times the essential fat, and anywhere from 4 to 6 times the amount of calcium as the processed product below. The trumpeted addition of all or most of the vitamins you "need" in quantities equal to or exceeding your "total" daily requirements is a sorry sham. Such advertising may give you a false sense of security about your vitamin intake:

- Because needs vary from individual to individual, no cereal product can legitimately claim to fulfill all your unique vitamin requirements.

- Many "enrichment" vitamins never reach your body tissues. Because of their fiber content, cereal manufacturers often promote their products as natural laxatives. Vitamins locked into roughage may only be yours on short-term loan.

- Since it is probable that not all vitamins are yet identified, artificial enrichment can hardly claim to restore all those nutrients that milling and processing remove.

- Because carbohydrates in the form of refined starch and refined sugar are practically the only ingredients of cereals, such products provide a built-in vitamin drain, which probably cannibalizes their own enrichment vitamins. With the poison comes the antidote.

You can safely conclude that the subtle, persuasive, and deceptive advertising of breakfast cereals is but another example of agribusiness' indifference to your nutritional good health and well-being.

From the Laboratory:
Additional Risks and Additive Hazards

Although the processor's sins against food are many, his most venal trespass involves the addition of alien, even toxic, substances to his products. The names of most of the 2,500 compounds commonly added to food are as foreign to the layman as Chinese verbs. You may need a Ph.D. in chemistry just to pronounce them, let alone evaluate their role in your diet.

One hundred forty pounds of additives are consumed per person per year. Because this amount represents the national average, your actual consumption may be higher or lower, depending on your relative intake of prepared and processed foods. Of the total ingested, 102 pounds is as sucrose, 15 pounds is as salt, and 13 pounds is as dextrose, a refined sugar found in corn syrup. Approximately 8 pounds of the remainder come from 30 common kitchen substances such as pepper, mustard, baking soda, and citric acid. Although the dangers of excessive sugar and salt intake are widely recognized as important factors in the development of such degenerative illnesses as diabetes and circulatory disorders, it is the remaining 2.1 pounds of additives—drawn from the food chemist's catalogue of more than 2,400 synthetic compounds—that create a major, unappreciated hazard to your health.

The various compounds included in this insidious 2.1 pounds of chemical cunning find frequent employment as colorants, preservatives, flavorings, thickeners, emulsifiers, dyes, detergents, ripeners, anti-oxidants, and bleaches. They may make a green tomato red, a thin soup hearty, a bland cheese zesty, or a perishable fruit impervious to decay. Many are simply poisonous. Sodium nitrates and nitrites are widely used color enhancers employed to "redden" sausage meats, corned beef, and bacon. Although toxic in and of themselves, they easily form cancer-causing *nitrosamines* on contact with other common food substances. Many FDA-approved colorants are implicated both in poisoning children and in inducing cancer in adults. Such food dyes as Blue #1 and #2, Citrus Red #2, Green #3, Orange B, Red #3 and #40, and Yellow #5 are liberally used to color candy, soft drinks, gelatin desserts, baked goods, pastry, hot dogs, and the skin of citrus fruits. Although some dyes are safer than others, you are wise to avoid all artificially colored foods since food labels do not indicate which dye is present and the dyed product is often of dubious nutritional value. Butylated hydroxytoluene (BHT), the common preservative included with breakfast cereals, dehydrated soups, vegetable oils, potato chips, and chewing gum, may cause cancer and can trigger allergic reactions among the young. Because of their relatively small body weight, their natural craving for sugar, and their vulnerability to the lure of processed-food advertising, children are generally the most susceptible to ill effects caused by additives. Impressive improvements in health have been obtained by eliminating these compounds from the diets of some hyperactive and otherwise emotionally disturbed youngsters.

Although not all food additives prove so dramatically and immediately injurious to health, little is known of their cumulative effects. Many cannot be broken down through normal metabolic processes. They tend to accumulate in your liver and other tissues. Even if such stored molecules are not themselves poisonous, concentrations built up over a lifetime may clog your tissues and eventually injure your health. There seems to be wisdom in avoiding food additives of all kinds, whenever possible. Why risk another bullet in today's game of nutritional Russian roulette?

From the Market: The Fresh Food Fallacy

Many Americans assume that fresh and unprocessed foods have eluded the grasp of the chemist's adulterating hand. Unfortunately, beautiful hypotheses are often slain by ugly facts. Virtually no crop plant or herd animal escapes some form of chemical manipulation between its time of planting or birth and its progress to your plate. A number of these chemical encounters are beneficial. Others clearly constitute a serious tampering or adulteration.

MEAT AND POULTRY

The "fresh" meat, poultry, and game you buy with confidence from your supermarket or butcher may be seriously compromised. An average of one pound in eight contains measurable quantities of agricultural drugs, antibiotics, pesticides, and/or environmental pollutants. Although many of these contaminants are thought to cause cancer, birth defects, and other ills in humans, their intrusion into the marketplace is not easily controlled. The law protects the meat wholesaler against impoundment of his product while samples undergo laboratory analysis. Because of the vast distances between pasture and market, the problems of preserving the nutritional integrity of meat are enormous. Despite the use of sophisticated refrigeration equipment, as much as 15 percent of the beef and pork that arrives in urban centers has undergone spoilage. Although the law requires that such meat be destroyed, in practice some of it is restored to normal color and aroma through the use of such colorants and deodorants as sodium sulfate. Although you cannot easily identify which cut of steak, loin of pork, or breast of chicken is chemically contaminated or nutritionally depleted, you can be sure that some of the meat and poultry you eat is less than pure, fresh, and unprocessed.

FRUITS AND VEGETABLES

Sun-ripened fruits and vegetables plucked and eaten from the branch or stalk are undoubtedly rich sources of natural energy, vitamins, and minerals. Life in high-rise apartment buildings and suburban villas places a considerable barrier between you and the orchard or garden. Agribusiness has the means to satisfy your yearning for "fresh" produce throughout the year. They involve the very chemical intrusion and loss of nourishment that fresh-food enthusiasts wish to avoid. Because the moment of ripeness is fleeting, most fruits and vegetables are harvested long before they are mature. Picked while "green," they lack many of the final vitamins they would have if allowed to ripen naturally. Since the growing season doesn't coincide with the prime economic demand of the winter months, preservation is essential. To prevent decay, stored fruits and vegetables are subjected to a host of chemical fumigants, retardants, preservatives, and anti-sprouting compounds. Prior to the ideal marketing moment, the half-ripened produce is propelled to artificial maturity with the help of chemical stimulants. To prevent natural dehydration, shriveling, and wizening, apples, cucumbers, and melons may be waxed. To create an appropriate color intensity, tomatoes, olives, and some lemons, oranges, and other citrus fruits may be dyed. To prevent discoloration, sulfur dioxide and sodium sulfate may be applied to apricots, apples, and potatoes. These techniques are as ingenious as they are deceptive.

It is difficult to know whether the fruits or vegetables you purchase in plastic-wrapped cardboard trays are genuinely "fresh" or somehow chemically contaminated or nutritionally impoverished. Although vigorous washing and scrubbing may be a good antidote to the former, assessment of the latter is virtually impossible. Consider and pity the poor potato. When dug from the ground in the fall, it contains a rich supply of vitamin C. By the spring its content of the vitamin falls to one quarter of the original and by the summer virtually all of the C is lost. In apples, similar concentrations of the vitamin fall to about one third of the original value after two to three months. Green vegetables suffer even greater losses. But because of clever methods of storage and preservation, the supermarket potato, apple, or green vegetable will look just the same in June as it did the previous September.

From the Executive Suite: Profit before Principle

A general decline in the quality of American food is undeniable. Much of the responsibility can be laid at the door of agribusiness and the occupants of its executive suites. A very few corporate executives wield tremendous power over America's agricultural riches, her nutritional well-being, and ultimately, her good health. Because primary concern is with profit rather than the principle of public welfare, these nutritional magnates have encouraged farming practices that pollute the land and slowly poison man. They have fostered the zeal of the food chemist and turned him into a kind of white-coated Dr. Strangelove whose crowning achievement will be the fabrication of an artificial apple. They have consistently approved the subtle cheapening of food with the substitution of calorierich and vitamin-poor oils, fats, and sugars for more nutritional ingredients. They have annually introduced more than a thousand new processed foods into the marketplace without adequate testing and controls. They have cynically seduced children and gullible adults into poor eating habits through incessant and persuasive advertising. They have falsely claimed virtue in the partial restoration of nutrients to foods they initially robbed of nutritional value. The indictment is severe and the "crimes" are heinous. None of them could have occurred without public cooperation, acceptance, and even approval.

CONSUMER COLLUSION IN THE DECLINE AND FALL OF THE AMERICAN DIET

European visitors to these shores often express amazement at the quantity, variety, and eye-appeal of American food. Their praise is usually tempered by disappointment that the visual promise is belied by blandness and absence of taste. After years of enervated foods, the American palate is numb. It no longer protects the individual from inferior food and poor eating habits.

The Lure of Convenience Foods

The crowded schedules and rapid pace of contemporary life leave little time for the careful preparation and leisurely consumption of food. Americans are generally willing to sacrifice their digestive systems to any vaguely palatable food product that promises to save even a few minutes in the kitchen or dining room. Cold cereals, breakfast squares, frozen orange juice, luncheon meats, commercial pastry, dried soups, TV dinners, canned goods, instant puddings, frozen vegetables, pre-cooked meats, gelatin desserts, package mixes, and the like are staple items in a typical diet. Each has a nutritionally richer and tastier natural counterpart. Yet the national preference is for the "convenience" alternatives because they "save time." Such savings are illusory. They sacrifice taste and bodily health while ensuring a major loss of time through a measurably shortened life.

Aesthetics vs. Rational Nutritional Choices

Even if you are a responsible consumer who does not succumb to the lure of convenience foods, you are apt to be duped by qualities in fresh foods that have little or nothing to do with their nutritional endowment. The reddest steak, the brightest orange, the most colorful tomato, and the plumpest apple are the prized purchases of the discriminating shopper. That food colorants, deodorizers, preservatives, dyes, and waxes may confer those "special" qualities on prime meat and produce rarely occurs to the consumer. How can it when there are no content labels affixed to fresh foods? Indeed, the public quest for "colorful, juicy, firm, and plump" products is well known to food producers who pander to these tastes in their selection of strains of fruit, vegetable, and farm animal that will satisfy these demands. That such desired characteristics have little to do with nutritional value is a sad reality. In fact, you are apt to be more critical of the dietary quality of the products you buy for your pet dog or cat than you are of the food that you purchase for yourself.

The Crime of the Cook

That you can number a civilization's diseases by

counting its cooks is an exaggeration, but it is undoubtedly true that many of the nutritional riches that enter the kitchen never reach the plate. Different methods for preparing and cooking food can do much to preserve or destroy essential nutrients, particularly vitamins and minerals. The cook who rapidly steams fresh vegetables and serves them when crisp and firm preserves most of the original nutrients. The cook who pre-soaks the same vegetables and boils or simmers them slowly until soft leaves many of the original vitamins in the pot. To ensure a minimum loss of vitamins and minerals, it is wise to follow a number of simple cooking rules.

- *Use fresh food in preference to processed alternatives.* Garden peas provide a typical illustration. If canned, more than 80 percent of the vitamin C content is lost in the commercial blanching, sterilizing, and soaking processes. If frozen, about 60 percent of the vitamin C content is lost in the blanching, freezing, and thawing processes. Fresh peas, if not pre-soaked, should retain their original vitamin C content. Typical cooking reduces levels of C by about half, so that fresh peas retain about 50 percent of the vitamin when eaten, canned peas about 6 percent, and frozen peas about 17 percent.

- *Use a minimum amount of water in cooking.* Meat that is rapidly broiled or sautéed will, for example, contain an average of 50 percent more of its original vitamins than the same meat slowly boiled in water to a state of "well-doneness."

- *Cook for a minimum period of time.* High temperature for a short period does the least vitamin damage.

- *Avoid storing cooked foods before serving.*

THE SIREN SONG OF A BALANCED DIET

That a balanced diet provides ideal nourishment has long been a fundamental article of faith among the high priests and priestesses of nutrition. Although such a diet is not typical of animals in Nature, the basic notion has surface appeal. You would seem to have the greatest probability of achieving an optimal intake of all necessary nutrients by drawing upon a wide variety of different foods from diverse sources. In urging this "shotgun" approach to food selection, dietary specialists tacitly admit that nutrition is not an exact science. In the absence of fixed laws and principles, the nutritional goal of a balanced diet is as alluring as it is confounding.

The Basic Four and Why They Don't Ensure Adequate Nutrition

According to the gospel of a balanced diet, the nutritional good life results when your diet combines and balances food drawn from four basic nutrient categories. These include:

Fruits and Vegetables   Dairy Products
 (Yellow and Green)
Meat, Fish, and Poultry   Grains and Cereals

In theory, an evenhanded selection of foods from these four classes should provide all necessary proteins, carbohydrates, essential fats, vitamins, minerals, and any yet-to-be-identified food elements that your body may need. In practice, this approach can probably ensure an ample intake of necessary food calories. It has little relevance to the adequate ingestion of vitamins, minerals, and other food elements. Even if impervious to the modern mania for prepared and processed foods, you might achieve a fine caloric balance by relying on the basic four and still be inadequately nourished. The reasons are many—

● *Nutritional Inequality within Food Classes.* A commercial cupcake and one serving of fresh, cooked lima beans provide a roughly equivalent number and distribution of protein, fat, and carbohydrate calories. The differences in vitamin and mineral values are enormous. In preferring steak to pork or liver, you retain approximate caloric parity, but deprive yourself of rich vitamin and mineral resources.

● *Impoverishment in Preparation.* Cooking does little to alter the protein, fat, or carbohydrate content of foods. Different preparation methods may either minimally affect or virtually destroy vitamin and mineral stores.

● *Nutritional Variability Results from Differences in Growth and Delivery.* Soil depletion, climatic adversity, transportation, and storage minimally alter the caloric content of most fresh foods. Where caloric values fluctuate, as in the fat content of milk and butter, farmers must supplement their products with enrichment calories. No similar addition is required for vitamins and minerals, which are most vulnerable to loss and depletion.

The widespread introduction of refined and processed products in recent decades further undermines the balanced diet concept. Although contemporary foods retain measurable and predictable amounts of protein, carbohydrate, and fat, chemical and physical manipulation plays havoc with their vitamin and mineral stores. Americans now consume *thirty fewer pounds* of fresh fruits and fresh vegetables per person per year than they did in 1950. Frozen, canned, bottled, and pre-cooked substitutes yield equivalent caloric values but dramatically reduced levels of essential vitamins and minerals. Wheat, cereals, and rice have become vitamin thieves through refinement. Processed cheeses, artificial creamers, manufactured yogurts, and other novel dairy products are apt to be rich in calories but poor in vitamins and minerals. A similar litany of caloric richness and vitamin impoverishment applies to most modern food alternatives found in each category of the Basic Four. Reliance on a conscientiously "balanced" diet may assure you of an abundant caloric subsidy. It does little to guarantee an adequate, equally essential, income of vitamins and minerals.

You Can't Count Vitamins as You Count Calories

At one time or another most Americans make a conscious effort to systematically gain or lose weight. Although the national physique-altering craze annually spawns thousands of dietary schemes, supplements, stimulants, and suppressants, all such programs and products represent elaborate, often bizarre, variations on a simple nutritional theme. One pound of body tissue is roughly equivalent to 4,000 calories of food energy. If your metabolism requires 2,500 calories of input for maintenance, a daily consumption of 1,500 calories will shed a pound of flesh in 4 days while an intake of 3,000 calories will predictably add a pound in 8. Because the energy content of most nutrients can be accurately measured and remains unaffected by variability in growing conditions, handling, processing, and cooking, product labels and standardized charts give a reliable account of the caloric content of most fresh or prepared foods. How convenient it would be if vitamin and mineral resources could be similarly identified, measured, and counted.

Over the past fifty years chemists have evolved various techniques for estimating the vitamin and mineral concentrations in different substances. Their methods, called assays, offer differing degrees of scientific reliability. Greatest precision and accuracy results in measuring the vitamin and mineral content of manufactured products for use as food supplements. These include the familiar single or multiple vitamin (or multimineral) capsule, tablet, liquid, or drop. Certainty is less assured with techniques designed to measure nutrient levels in your blood, lymph, and other body tissue.

Assays of food prove unreliable because of differences in soil quality, peculiar growing conditions, storage, transportation, processing, and cooking. The values derived from these analyses tend to overestimate the actual vitamin or mineral amounts you obtain from your food. The laboratory assay of raw carrots registers a high concentration of the vitamin A precursor known as carotene. It neglects the fact that the rich stores of this vitamin are

locked into cells that you cannot digest. Most of the carotene passes through your body bound in roughage. The
same is true for the indigestible form of carotene in cabbage, the niacin in many cereals, and the iron in fresh
spinach. Although most of the B-complex vitamins are
drained from asparagus after steaming or boiling, the food
analyst's chart records vitamin B levels for the vegetable
as if cooking did not ordinarily occur. Seasonal variations
may lower the vitamin E content of milk and butter by
more than half, yet published assays reflect the high concentrations of peak summer months. The potato, whose
vitamin C content is highest at harvest in the fall and
virtually depleted by the following summer, is typically
assayed in September rather than July. The vitamin A
concentration lost to nitrate preservatives in meat is no
more reckoned with than the large losses of A, C, and
B-complex vitamins lost through the usual cooking of red,
green, and yellow vegetables. In sum, standardized vitamin and mineral charts suggest that foods contain improb-
ably high amounts of these essential nutrients. Since you
cannot know the unique history of the food you buy and
eat, it is impossible for you to count your dietary vitamins
and minerals as you count your calories.

The Nutritionist's Conundrum

The Food and Drug Administration insists that the
"average diet is adequate for the needs of all healthy
Americans." This contention is generally confirmed by
prominent food analysts, statisticians, and dietary plan-
ners. Their figures persuasively argue that when the nation's gross production of food calories, vitamins, and
minerals is divided by the number of her citizens,
the amounts of each nutrient available *per person* far exceed the nutritional needs of any "average" individual.
These same food experts express profound puzzlement at
contrary conclusions drawn from nutritional surveys conducted by the United States Department of Agriculture.
These latter evaluations, which deal with real people

rather than abstract statistics, indicate that the quality of the American diet is rapidly deteriorating.

According to USDA assessments, 60 percent of the population enjoyed a "good" diet in 1955, while only 50 percent achieved a similar intake by 1965. Deficiencies in protein, calcium, iron, and vitamins A, B_1, B_2, and C are common. It is typical of this general dietary decline that an estimated 80 million Americans suffer from measurable vitamin A depletion, while as many as 25 million have no body stores of this essential vitamin at all. The enormous gap between the rosy nutritional picture painted by the FDA and the alarming reality depicted by the Department of Agriculture has its origin in many causes. Previously discussed agricultural practices, modern food handling and processing techniques, personal and corporate economics, public ignorance and indifference, changing lifestyles, and overly confident assessments of the nutritive worth of contemporary foods all may be held accountable. The implications for you, your children, and your grandchildren are chilling.

MALNUTRITION KNOWS NO CLASS DISTINCTIONS

There is cold comfort and considerable error in assuming that malnutrition stalks none but the poor and underprivileged. Inadequate foods and injurious eating habits are as typical of the penthouse, boardroom, and suburban household as they are of the nation's urban and Appalachian ghettos.

Upper Income Undernourishment

The corporate executive who breakfasts on refined cereal, processed fruit juice, and multiple cups of coffee; who lunches on three martinis, a few bites of pre-cooked steak with sodden vegetables; and who sups on more alcohol, caffeine, and a reheated meal is a familiar figure. He is committing slow but sure nutritional suicide. His equally identifiable wife may ride a dietary roller coaster with weeks of excessive eating followed by months of self-recriminatory and self-imposed fasting. Her cyclic vacillation between feast and famine places abnormal stress on her metabolism and invites premature aging and degenerative ills. In conforming to peer pressure, the adolescent daughter of this affluent couple may fashionably starve herself into a state of *anorexia,* or appetite suppression, while her teenage brother may rely on "junk" foods, quick energy snacks, and other processed products to fuel his metabolic fires. Similar dietary mayhem is common among unmarried professionals, divorced persons, and "swinging singles" who find little time or motivation to eat with care. Even more debilitating habits typify the elderly, whose diets are apt to suffer because of straitened finances, reduced taste perception, dental problems, mental depression, and chronic diseases that make marketing and the proper preparation of food difficult.

The High Cost of Nutritional Ignorance

Although the question of why Johnny can't read, write, or do his sums is a properly burning educational issue, it masks an equally important question about why he is a nutritional illiterate.

Modern biology teaching concentrates on the theoretical beauties and complexities of cellular biochemistry at the expense of practical learning about how dietary choices affect these fascinating processes. Health and hygiene courses are second-class curricular citizens, the traditional objects of student indifference and derision. An era sensitive to legitimate demands for full equality between men and women downgrades the educational importance of studies in home economics, society's one reliable source of nutritionally knowledgeable individuals. Attaining equivalent ignorance between the sexes constitutes a pyrrhic victory for women and a sad loss for humanity.

Dietary recklessness is often the domain of well-educated and well-to-do segments of society. The fashionable weight-loss diet is an almost certain route to vitamin depletion and metabolic misery. How many of the college graduates who embark on liquid protein regimens realize their risk of death from potassium depletion? How many associate high protein intake with vitamin A deficiency and its subsequent symptoms of itching and vision impairment? How many know that the crotchety ill humor of reduced food intake is more probably the result of vitamin B starvation than hunger? How many realize the dangers of failing to meet their vitamin needs over prolonged periods? Academic excellence is no guarantee of nutritional wisdom.

You Are the Product of Your Dietary History

Every American over fifty years of age lived through the Great Depression, when the diets of about 90 percent of the nation's families achieved only marginal subsistence levels. Because there is impressive evidence that even temporary nutritional deprivation has profound and long-term effects on your health, there is considerable speculation that the alarming increase in degenerative ills in modern times may have its origins in the all-but-forgotten past. Support for this idea comes from studies of prisoners of war, displaced persons, and concentration camp victims who were subjected to dietary atrocities. After years of restored nutritional abundance, many of these once-abused individuals still show signs of severe emotional depression, lack of vitality, and susceptibility to disease. Although the conventional impulse is to ascribe their problems to psychological causes, large numbers respond favorably to massive doses of vitamins and minerals. Remission of symptoms seems a function of continuous supplementation. Evidently, past vitamin depletion can elevate present metabolic needs on a continuing basis. In theory, milder forms of deprivation, resulting from poor adolescent eating habits, fad diets, food taboos, or the temporary stresses of illness, may effect a similar and permanent elevation in vitamin requirements.

Air increasingly polluted by industrial poisons and automobile exhausts, cigarettes, alcohol, processed foods, hypertension, infections, and drugs such as aspirin, steroids, oral contraceptives, antibiotics, and sulfanilamides all assault your vitamin reserves. Digestive tract disorders such as diarrhea, colitis, liver and gall bladder malfunction, and/or the use of laxatives tend to reduce your ability to absorb dietary vitamins. That the vitamin content of your food is deteriorating at a time when your demands are probably increasing is alarming. You are not only what you eat, but have become and will continue to become what you have eaten.

CAN YOU GET ALL THE VITAMINS YOU NEED WITH YOUR KNIFE AND FORK?

Conventional medical wisdom answers this question in the affirmative, and much can be favorably said for increased attention to the quality and quantity of what you eat. Although vitamin-impoverished foods are typical of the age, most Americans still achieve input adequate to avoid outright deficiency diseases. That you may wonder about the differences between "adequate" and "optimal" ingestion is logical. The FDA and more conventional representatives of the medical establishment have little to say about the matter. Other highly respected scientists, medical authorities, and government agencies offer compelling evidence that vitamin concentrations sufficient to prevent deficiency diseases fall far short of levels necessary for maximum good health and biochemical function.

Even if your goal is simply to meet the suggested daily allowances of vitamins proposed by the FDA, it is difficult to see how contemporary calorie-rich and vitamin-poor foods can meet such quotas. Avoidance of all processed products, careful selection of fresh foods, minimal cooking, and a return to many once-favored and vitamin-rich staples such as pork, yeast, liver, fresh fruits, fresh vegetables, whole grains, honey, and unrefined oils *might* ensure an adequate vitamin intake at the dining table. Unfortunately, the nature of modern life makes such heroic measures inconvenient if not totally impractical. To supplement a calorically rich and nutritionally impoverished diet with known quantities of vitamins and minerals will help the body metabolize its "empty" food calories while minimizing the biochemical insults of an increasingly contaminated environment.

2

Vitamin Deficiencies:
Myth or Reality?

Disease is the retribution of an outraged nature.

— BALLOU

Because your body cannot synthesize the vitamins necessary to regulate its intricate biochemical processes, your diet must continuously supply them. Although some fat-soluble varieties can be stored, the water-soluble majority rapidly disappear with the daily ebb and flow of body fluids. As supplies of a particular vitamin are exhausted, increasingly severe and horrifying disease is the result. Should the missing nutrient not be replenished, gradual debilitation and eventual death will follow.

VITAMIN DEFICIENCIES: THE SHADOWS OF FORGOTTEN ANCESTORS

The inexorable link between vitamin depletion and disease has counted as a major cause of death through the ages, regularly decimating whole armies, navies, and nations. Its insidious cause and effect explain many of the dramatic, otherwise inexplicable, turns of event that have permanently altered the course of human history.

Egyptian hieroglyphics, incised into temple walls more than 5,000 years ago, speak through time and warn the modern reader to avoid certain blindness by consuming the liver of cattle, oxen, or other beasts. Cave paintings from ancient China depict crippled men, women, and children, the bent and twisted victims of evident rickets, or vitamin D deprivation. Physicians from the Golden Age of Greece write of cities with whole populations unaccountably suffering from weakness, bleeding gums, and baffling bruises, the unmistakable symptoms of scurvy, or vitamin C deficiency.

Although such pitiable descriptions are common relics of antiquity, a similar legacy is part and parcel of our more contemporary heritage. From the hundreds of thousands who embarked on medieval crusades, but a few tens of thousands survived. The celebrated but sightless beggars, or mendicants, who wandered over Europe with marvellous tales of the Holy Land, paid for their piety with blindness probably caused by a lack of the vitamin A essential for vision. Chronicles of less fortunate pilgrims provide vivid descriptions of frequent slow and agonizing death. Although explained as the will of God by the faithful, most typify the final and mortal throes of scurvy, rickets, beri beri (lack of vitamin B_1), or pellagra (lack of vitamin B_3).

Similar sufferings haunt the pages of naval history as seafarers have traditionally had more to fear from the specter of scurvy than from the terrors of tempest or cannon. The scourge cost Vasco da Gama two thirds of his crew during his fifteenth-century search for a passage to India. Lifeless hulks, the morbid treasure-laden remnants of once-proud Spanish galleons, were common sights on calm sixteenth-century Caribbean waters. Scurvy claimed 626 lives on Sir George Anson's eighteenth-century voyage around the world. Richard Walter, one of Anson's lieutenants, recorded the dread progress of this most baffling disease:

Soon after our passing *Streights Le Maire,* the scurvy began to make its appearance among us; and our long continuance at sea, the fatigue we underwent, and the various disappointments we met with, had occasioned its spreading to such a degree, that at the latter end of April there were but a few on board, who were not in some degree afflicted with it, and in that month, no less than forty-three died of it on board the *Centurion.* But though we thought that the distemper had then risen to an extraordinary height, and were willing to hope that as we advanced to the northward its malignity would abate, yet we found, on the contrary, that in the month of May we lost nearly double that number: And as we did not get to land till the middle of June, the mortality went on increasing, and the disease extended itself so prodigiously, that after the loss of above two hundred men, we could not at last muster more than six foremast men in a watch capable of duty.

Although the effectiveness of citrus fruits as scurvy-preventives had been demonstrated as early as 1757, it took the British Admiralty forty years to mandate the inclusion of limes in a sailor's diet. Its albeit tardy order was sufficient to fortify the English navy and thwart Napoleon's grand design for the invasion of Great Britain. "Limeys," immune to scurvy, could withstand many months of blockade duty, while their vulnerable French counterparts were regularly enfeebled and had to be replaced within weeks.

Although such nutritional horror stories may seem the stuff of history books, they have continued to exert a grim hand in shaping the recent past, the present, and the future. Widespread incidence of pellagra among the corn-fed, vitamin B_3-deprived armies of the Confederacy contributed measurably to the success of Union forces during the Civil War. In this century, alarming numbers of outright or marginal deficiency diseases were revealed by the Universal Draft of 1940 and produced dramatic government intervention into America's agricultural and food industry practices. Today, the nutritional nightmares of scurvy, beri beri, rickets, and other severe deficiency diseases continue to mock Third World countries, sapping their vitality, causing untold suffering, and preventing the full realization of their vast human potential.

NUTRITIONAL DISEASE AND THE GERM DOCTORS

The second half of the nineteenth century was a period rich in scientific, medical, and intellectual ferment. It bore ripe fruit for mankind as it provided a rational explanation for his place in Nature, healed many of his most terrible diseases, and explored the mysteries of his psyche. While Darwin published his radical Theory of Evolution in England, Freud probed the human mind and developed his ingenious theory of personality in Vienna. Pasteur in France, Koch in Germany, and Metchnikoff in Russia together formulated the Germ Theory of Disease, which explained the causes and produced the cures for many epidemic disorders. All three theories were the product of an exquisite synthesis of research data and idea. All three had profound implications for understanding the nature and function of vitamins.

The discovery that microbes caused such rampant diseases as smallpox, tuberculosis, and purpureal fever fired the imagination of scientists and spurred their search for micro-organisms as the *agents provocateurs* of epidemic sickness. The infectious nature of malaria, yellow fever, and influenza was rapidly established and reinforced the belief that bacteria, protozoa, and viruses would ultimately prove the source of all human illness. Although the Germ Theory continues viable in unlocking the mysteries of disease and provides a sound rationale for seeking the causes of cancer among viruses, its overzealous application can color or confound research thinking. Not all diseases, even ones of an apparently epidemic nature, result from infection.

•   •   •

In 1911 a young Polish biochemist named Casimir Funk was deeply engaged in studying four widespread maladies: scurvy, beri beri, rickets, and pellagra. Despite their occurrence in epidemic proportions, research scientists had been unable to link them with any ultimate infectious agent or demonstrate their capacity for contagion. Working independently and against the grain of orthodox thinking, Funk gradually evolved a theory to explain the nature, cause, and cure for these dread but elusive disorders. Combining and synthesizing evidence provided by hundreds of researchers, he reasoned that victims of these maladies must share a common nutritional deficiency that disrupts normal metabolic function. Although carbohydrates, proteins, and fats were the only recognized nutrients in food at the time, Funk proposed that a fourth and equally essential category was ordinarily present, but in such minute quantities that it had previously escaped detection. He gave the name "vitamines" to this hypothetical group of micronutrients and predicted that the absence of any one from a person's diet would cause serious, if not lethal, disruption of body processes.

The implications of Funk's alternative to the Germ Theory of Disease were quickly appreciated and seized upon by the worldwide scientific community. In four subsequent decades, tremendous research energy and talent were expended on finding, isolating, and synthesizing these occult nutrients. Just as pioneering Germ Theory research had yielded scientific gold, pursuit of the vitamins proved rewarding. The vitamins—whose absence causes scurvy, pellagra, beri beri, rickets, some forms of blindness, certain anemias, and other deficiency diseases —were discovered, refined, and related to normal metabolic function. The work took many years and thousands of chemists from many countries. Successful identification, isolation, or synthesis of a particular vitamin often generated a Nobel Prize or similar recognition for the successful research chemist.

By 1940 enough was known to suggest that certain vitamins are necessary to every cell in the body and that all are essential for the maintenance of life. With the clear establishment of minimum concentrations necessary to prevent deficiency diseases, theoreticians eagerly speculated that increased vitamin consumption might confer important health benefits through improved metabolic function. Optimistic reports in the scientific literature led to a lavish expenditure of research time and money in a manner not dissimilar to today's extravagant "War on Cancer." The use of vitamin therapies became rapidly fashionable, fed by inflated reports of dramatic cures for an increasing number of diseases.

By 1950 early scientific enthusiasm had evaporated in the teeth of apparently negative evidence. Medical researchers—intent on discovering another group of "wonder drugs" equivalent to antibiotics and sulfanilamides—were thwarted in their diligent efforts to bend supplementary vitamins into powerful therapeutic tools capable of *curing* such then dread diseases as polio. The best evidence—generated through undeniably careful research, close observation, and repeated testing—*seemed* irrefutable: Vitamins are essential to life. By maintaining adequate dietary concentrations, all of the deficiency disorders can be avoided. Increasing intake beyond the levels adequate to avoid such diseases has little discernible effect on any other disease.

To members of the medical and scientific establishment, the time, labor, and money spent in postwar vitamin studies seemed wasted. Their sense of futility resulted in a generally negative attitude toward any further expenditure for vitamin research. Other lines of scientific inquiry seemed more remunerative. Alas, in their haste to uncover rapid-fire, miracle-working agents for curing acute disease, few thought about or were willing to investigate the long-term use of vitamins as *preventive* rather than curative factors in human health. Betting on Aesop's hare rather than his tortoise is a natural human impulse—even among research scientists, who are supposed to be above such mortal failings. However, such behavior more than twenty-five years ago is not surprising in light of contemporary attitudes among medical men who continue to view "preventive" medicine as a matter of early *diagnosis* rather than the actual contravention of disease *before* it occurs.

VITAMIN DEFICIENCIES TODAY: CONTENTION, CONTROVERSY, AND CONFUSION

Although vitamin malnutrition continues to wreak havoc among the impoverished countries of the world, the incidence of vitamin-depletion diseases in the industrialized nations is relatively rare. Agricultural abundance, a high standard of living, and sophisticated medical practices have virtually eliminated the perils of such killing disorders as pellagra, scurvy, and beri beri.

Parroting the scientific and medical consensus established in the early 1950s, the FDA insists that the typical American diet is adequate for the vitamin needs of healthy individuals. In the ongoing controversy that surrounds vitamin use and abuse, the word "adequate" is a major and fundamental source of contention and confusion.

Based on the assumption that genuine vitamin insufficiency produces only depletion diseases and the observation that vitamin-depletion disorders are nonexistent in the United States, the logic of the FDA and its principal allies is unassailable. To contemporary advocates of preventive medicine, any thinking that equates vitamin adequacy with the simple prevention of devastating clinical illness is antediluvian. They argue that such amounts are woefully inadequate if an individual is to enjoy optimal health. They propose vitamin ingestion at levels that radically exceed the current recommendations of Federal agencies and far outstrip those concentrations employed in postwar vitamin research.

THE GREAT VITAMIN DEFICIENCY DEBATE: A CASE FOR THE PLAINTIFF

Critics of the FDA interpretation of national vitamin needs generally integrate their specific charges into a broader indictment of the official health-care policy and modern medical practice. Their allegations are severe, but their evidence is formidable. Although far from conclusive, these arguments cannot be dismissed with impunity.

Modern Medical Muddleheadedness

That too many doctors have killed too many people with too many drugs and too much surgery is not an idea drawn from the pages of *1984* or *Brave New World,* but a grim opinion that is achieving widespread public recognition and stimulating massive criticism of the medical profession. Reports that more than 30,000 people will needlessly die this year from sensitivity to antibiotics or that as many as 50 percent of all surgical procedures are unnecessary cause justifiable alarm. Such statistics gain particular credibility as major health insurance plans now urge their subscribers to seek a second and corroborative medical opinion—at company expense—before obediently submitting to the knife.

Distrust of the scalpel and the prescription pad are identifiable symptoms of a growing dissatisfaction with once-revered principles and practices of the medical profession. The nationwide preoccupation with physical fitness, passion for jogging, pursuit of "health" foods, and concern about pollution reflect a gut understanding that the prevalent diseases of modern times have their origin in a lifetime of injurious living and eating habits in an increasingly poisonous environment. Concern for ensuring good health *while still healthy* reveals an intuitive knowledge that failure of the human body doesn't happen overnight or at any particular, fixed, or given moment. It indicates a passionate desire to prevent the degenerative, crippling, and humiliating illnesses currently typical of old age. People increasingly reject medical practice that is powerless to intervene in their personal health until after a dread and debilitating disease has taken hold of the body. Popular impulse demands a preventive approach to health care. It is a sentiment the American medical establishment cannot long choose to ignore.

Declining Public Health

Until the early 1960s national life expectancy continued to climb and promised to fulfill the Biblical model of a full threescore years and ten. Prospects for a longer life were widely publicized as evidence for the superiority of American medicine and the American way of life. Much of the congratulatory tumult and shouting has died during the past fifteen years.

Today, our national life expectancy ranks eighteenth among all nations. Our betters include not only the socialized states of northern Europe but a number of Iron Curtain countries and some less-than-wealthy Mediterranean republics as well. Although such a statistic seems shocking, it does not reveal the ominous face of things to come. While the senior citizen is apt to hold his statistical place among counterparts in other nations, prognostications for his children and grandchildren are bleak.[1] The current death rate for an American male between 40 and 50 years of age is the second highest among all industrial nations. His son of 20 will predictably be outlived by men of the same age in 37 other countries. His daughter of 20 will have a shorter lifetime than her contemporaries in 23 other countries. Her unborn children now have a 150 percent greater probability of becoming vulnerable low-birth-weight babies than they did 10 years ago. Their statistical chances for surviving infancy are greater in at least a dozen other lands. Although American life expectancy statistics now compare unfavorably with those of other

1. According to the Surgeon General, the death rate for young people 15 to 24 years of age grew by 11 percent between 1960 and 1979. In 1978—the last year for which complete data are available—the rate jumped by nearly 3 percent.

nations—despite our enormous fiscal investment in health care—they promise to deteriorate further and threaten to become unconscionable.

Even more appalling than a shrinking life span is the current erosion in the quality of life and health among the living. More than 24 million Americans now suffer from chronic and disabling disease. Although suffering and impairment does not necessarily affect their longevity, it becomes a distressing fact of personal life and weakens the fabric of national well-being. It surely undermines public confidence in the medical profession's ability to cope with the health problems of the age.

Technical Wizardry and Black Bag Impotence

It is ironic that a national decline in health and loss of professional esteem should plague medical practitioners at a time when they have acquired unparalleled skills and equipment for the diagnosis and treatment of disease. Increasingly sophisticated drugs, life-support apparatus, surgical devices, and laboratory procedures fill the doctor's little black bag to overflowing. He is awesomely armed with heroic techniques superbly designed for dramatic intervention into the very life processes of a body in crisis.

That a medical doctor's tools and training should focus on acute disruptions of the metabolism is both logical and necessary. His assistance is traditionally sought during times of severe bodily crisis. Diagnostic techniques and therapeutic measures capable of identifying and relieving critical disease are his principal articles of faith and instruments of practice. By his Hippocratic oath he is primarily bound to healing sickness.

In its commitment to the curative ideal, American medicine has unquestionably erected the most complex and sophisticated medical apparatus in the world. Its hospitals, support personnel, and technologies are without peer. Its doctors are the most rigorously and exhaustively trained. Whether this lavish curative edifice is entirely relevant to contemporary health problems is open to question.

Symptoms of the Times

Although the records are sketchy and far from complete, characteristic and predominant diseases can apparently be associated with particular historical eras or epochs. During the Middle Ages, death from bubonic plague, the sweating sickness, or dropsy was common. Consumption (tuberculosis) and tertian fevers superceded these disorders in subsequent periods, while infectious diseases have until recently been the primary cause of modern mortality. With the discovery of antibiotics and viral vaccines, the predominance of contagious illnesses gave way to a group of disorders that differ from their predecessors. They are essentially degenerative rather than infectious in nature. They tend to develop slowly over many years rather than manifest themselves suddenly and dramatically. They generally cannot be "cured" with the finality and certainty characteristic of their infectious cousins.

Heart and circulatory disorders, the many varieties of cancer, and diabetes (or conditions resulting from diabetic complications) constitute the principal lethal diseases of modern industrial societies. Non-lethal arthritis and rheumatism are similarly prevalent and share many characteristics with their killing counterparts. Twenty years may elapse between exposure to carcinogens, or cancer-causing agents, and the appearance of clinical symptoms of the disease. Hyperglycemia, or elevated levels of blood sugar, usually predates the full manifestations of diabetes by a decade or more. Fatty deposits or plaques, which reduce the size of blood vessels, usually precede heart attacks and other cardiovascular accidents by similar periods, as do the profound changes in bone structure leading to arthritis. Current medical methods for recognizing and controlling *incipient* cancer, diabetes, coronaries, arthritis, and strokes are comparatively primitive. Available drugs, where they exist, only relieve symptoms of an imminent disorder and generally do not attack fundamental causes leading to disease. Some, like the oral insulins used to control pre-diabetic conditions, may actually hasten expression of the overt illness. Once a heart attack occurs, a malignancy develops, or other certain clinical symptoms of a degenerative disorder appear, the physician achieves a greater measure of diagnostic and therapeutic certainty. Although many of his manipulative techniques undeniably ameliorate or relieve degenerative conditions, they often do not cure. They, too, tend to grapple with symptoms rather than causes. Often they produce such major physical or chemical disruption that victims may properly wonder whether the treatment isn't more terrible than the disease. Indeed, one may plausibly argue that the American doctor's overuse of the scalpel and prescription may not so much reflect a desire to line his pockets as a deep sense of frustration with the impotency of his elaborate skills and machinery in the face of contemporary degenerative illness.

Vitamin Deficiency and Degenerative Disease: Cause and Effect?

Preventing a disease, whether chronic or infectious, is obviously preferable to effecting its cure. Vaccines, which confer immunity to once-dread viral and bacterial illnesses, have retired many elaborate and costly treatment procedures to the medical dustbin. The appeal of discovering a microbial cause for contemporary degenerative illness and subsequently providing a protective inoculation for its prevention and a "magic bullet" for its cure has commanded almost unlimited research dollars and manhours in recent years. Failure to discover a viral origin for cancer, arthritis, and related disorders strongly suggests that a predilection for Germ Theory explanations of disease may have led the American research community down the proverbial garden path.

The most promising avenues of current inquiry and practice indicate that genetic, environmental, nutritional, and emotional factors are prime culprits in the mushrooming incidence of chronic ills. With few exceptions, substances that cause cancer in laboratory animals (certain insecticides, food additives, industrial wastes, nicotine, and caffeine, among others) will cause cancer in humans. Of more than 6,000 compounds tested, roughly 2,000 have proved carcinogenic. High dietary concentrations of refined sugar and carbohydrate in the modern diet clearly contribute to the development of diabetes. Poor physical conditioning, complicated by pollution, emotional stress, and diets rich in animal fat, is thought to make the body vulnerable to heart disease and circulatory disorders. The implications seem clear. Prevention of modern degenerative diseases will probably involve major and long-term modifications in American lifestyles, eating habits, and environmental quality. Major responsibility for necessary changes resides not so much with physicians and the medical establishment as with the individual and the public desire for good health.

Among the factors implicated in the development of chronic and debilitating diseases, nutritional malfeasance emerges as a *primus inter pares*, or a first among equals. The incidence of pre-clinical heart disorders, circulatory deterioration, and diabetes among young Americans has increased enormously in recent years. These symptoms of early disintegration and premature aging all appear before the four or five decades of stress and exposure to pollutants that once preceded such ills. That the general decline in the nutritive value of the national diet coincides with increased incidence of degenerative disease is undeniable. That vitamins, among all food elements, suffer most severely from the impoverishment of food is highly suggestive. Considerable evidence links less-than-optimal intake of these essential nutrients with the progressive development of degenerative illness.

SUB-CLINICAL VITAMIN DEFICIENCIES:
A UNIFIED THEORY OF DISEASE?

A life without vitamins is soon no life at all. Just as every cell in your body requires a regular supply of oxygen, each equally depends on a continuous source of the B-complex vitamins to utilize oxygen in the step-by-step release of stored energy from carbohydrate, fat, and protein. This sequential process, called cellular respiration, relies upon a specific enzyme for every stage of the conversion process. Instructions for the synthesis of each enzyme reside in the genetic code of master DNA and RNA molecules. They control the formation of protein portions of each enzyme from the pool of amino acids supplied by your diet. Before specific respiratory enzymes can function, they must chemically combine with a particular B-complex molecule. Essential supplies of these *co*-enzymes (vitamins) come from food, following digestion, absorption, and delivery by the bloodstream.

The numbers, or concentrations, of complete and functional respiratory enzymes in a cell depend on its supplies of vitamins and amino acids. If either or both are in short measure, respiration will continue, but with reduced efficiency and effectiveness. If either or both are depleted, respiration ceases and the cell dies. Complete exhaustion of amino acid reserves is unlikely since proteins are stored both in the body and in the cell itself. Far more vulnerable are the supplies of vitamin co-enzymes. Because they are water soluble and cannot be stored, a complete turnover of respiratory vitamins occurs within days. Vitamins A, D, and E are fat soluble and can be stored in body tissues. Although not required by every cell, they, too, act as co-enzymes and are essential to specific cells and tissues without which survival is impossible.

In its relentless quest to fulfill the metabolic needs of all its various cells, our body must maintain a continuous supply of all the various vitamins. Its nutritional marketing list invariably includes quantities[2] of—

THE WATER-SOLUBLE VITAMINS

Letter Designation	Common Name
B_1	Thiamin
B_2	Riboflavin
B_3	Niacin
B_6	Pyridoxine
B_{12}	Cobalamin
—	Folic Acid
—	Pantothenic Acid
—	Biotin
—	Choline
C	Ascorbic Acid

THE FAT-SOLUBLE VITAMINS

Letter Designation	Common Name
A	Retinol
D	Calciferol
E	Tocopherol
K	—

Because the human body is enormously resourceful, it can withstand biochemical assault and battery for decades without betraying any overt signs of suffering or damage. Although a crude and primitive machine by comparison, an automobile demonstrates a similar, though

---

2. Because they all act as respiratory fuels that release energy for use by a cell, biochemists often measure quantities of proteins, carbohydrates, and fats in terms of the *calories* of heat they generate. The water-soluble vitamins are described by metric units of *weight* in which 1 gram (g) = 1,000 milligrams (mg) = 1,000,000 micrograms (mcg or μg) = $\frac{1}{28}$ ounce. The fat-soluble varieties are categorized by their *chemical activity*, or potency, expressed in International Units (IU).

limited, resilience. It can run for a number of years on inferior fuels, lubricants, and electrolytes. That such abuse will have an immediate and obvious impact on a car's performance is uncertain. That it will produce excessive wear, tear, and a shortened driving life is without question. In a similar fashion, generations of human cells may function for decades with less-than-optimal enzyme concentrations resulting from an inadequate intake of vitamins. It may take years of such biochemical insult before the body revolts and the effects of such deprivation become obvious.

Vitamin Depletion or Vitamin Deficiency: A Case of Mistaken Identity?

Depletion diseases such as scurvy, beri beri, and pellagra only occur after the body's supplies of a particular vitamin are cut off and tissue stores are virtually exhausted. Such absolute deprivation causes acute metabolic disruptions, produces severe clinical symptoms, and threatens imminent death. Although medical schools train their students to recognize the classical symptoms of vitamin-depletion disorders, most modern doctors rarely encounter clear-cut clinical cases of such severe disease. Virtually everyone gets enough vitamins from his diet to prevent total cell and tissue depletion.

That most physicians cannot detect the signs of prolonged or intermittent vitamin insufficiency is a reality of modern medicine. An intake that is more than adequate to prevent a clinical depletion disease, like pellagra, but less than the cellular optimum, or ideal, manifests itself in subtle, variable, and confusing ways. Because their effects are not obvious or consistent, the symptoms of vitamin deprivation are often described as *sub-clinical.* Since many years may pass before such deficiencies are felt, there is often little apparent correlation between the eventual disease and its initial cause. To demonstrate that declining health, degenerative ills, and premature aging result from long-term sub-clinical vitamin deficiencies is not easy. It *is* easy to arbitrarily equate and confound vitamin *deficiency* with vitamin *depletion*. By blurring the distinctions between the two conditions, medical authorities can "prove" that vitamin "deficiencies" do not exist among Americans. To wit:

A) Scurvy results from a lack of vitamin C.
B) No one suffers from scurvy in this country.
C) Therefore, there is no lack of vitamin C in the U.S.A.

Unassailable reasoning with faulty premises does violence to the truth. That prolonged lack of ascorbic acid weakens the body's defenses and makes it vulnerable to infection is a fundamental, if not obvious, medical verity. One officially dies of pneumonia, not the chronic vitamin C deficiency which ultimately leads to death.

Sub-Clinical Ills

When supplies of a particular vitamin are entirely eliminated from the diet, obvious or clinical symptoms of insufficiency do not manifest themselves for weeks or months. While clinical signs of injury are absent, profound metabolic damage is occurring. Although normal biochemical processes continue until tissue stores of the vitamin are exhausted, derangement of essential molecular processes takes place as a state of depletion approaches. Usual function is impaired as alternative, less efficient metabolic pathways are activated or as the most vulnerable cells die, disintegrate, and release their stored vitamins for reuse by the still living tissue. Because the cells, tissues, and organs most susceptible to biochemical disruption are determined by individual genetic endowment and biochemical history, external symptoms of internal turmoil are apt to be subtle, variable, and confounding. Richard Walter, in his eighteenth-century description of scurvy, provides a still compelling and accurate account of the confusing and contradictory symptoms typical of a developing vitamin deficiency and depletion disorder.

This disease, so frequently attending all long voyages, and so particularly destructive to us, is surely the most singular and unaccountable of any that affects the human body. For its symptoms are inconstant and innumerable, and its progress and effects extremely irregular; for scarcely any two persons have the same complaints, and where there has been found some conformity in the symptoms, the order of their appearance has been totally different. However, it frequently puts on the form of many other diseases, and is therefore not to be described by any exclusive and infallible criterions.

Evidently, sub-clinical vitamin deficiencies strike any site where vitamin levels are in short supply and clearly develop in different individuals at different times and in different ways.

It is only after extended periods of total deprivation that the classical symptoms of a particular vitamin-depletion disease inevitably appear. It is this third and final stage of deficiency, or depletion, that is familiar to the modern medical doctor. It signals an imminent collapse of the body.

Although it is understandably difficult to find human subjects willing to expose themselves to the devastations of total vitamin depletion, a number of contemporary researchers have gathered statistically significant numbers of volunteers for the purpose. In a recent study of controlled vitamin B_1 depletion, it took from 5 to 10 days for evidence of sub-clinical cellular disruption to appear in all test subjects. This 100 percent variation between the initial dietary elimination of B_1 and the appearance of cellular injury—detectable only with sensitive laboratory techniques—is a function of biochemical individuality. Although the cells of all subjects showed signs of injury after 10 days, it wasn't until the 200th day of total B_1 abstinence that anyone began to actively experience the specific clinical symptoms of beri beri. During the 190-day interval, a period of sub-clinical deficiency, everyone suffered from increasing ill health. Symptoms ranged among weight loss, insomnia, appetite suppression, headache, malaise, irritability, and anxiety. None of these vague signs of distress developed at the same time or in the same sequence among the different volunteers.

Although the chances of completely and inadvertently excluding a particular vitamin from the modern diet are remote, it is quite probable that extended *sub-optimal* intake of one or more vitamins is typical of most Americans. Unique biochemical requirements, vitamin-poor foods, illness, pollution, and emotional stress are but a few of the factors that may lead to intake sufficient to prevent clinical disease but inadequate to prevent tissue deprivation and less-than-optimal cell function.

That most adults may suffer from the subtle and insidious effects of chronic vitamin deficiency is possible, even probable. Such deprivation may well account for the many vague symptoms of illness typical of modern life. It could explain much of the depression, malaise, and anxiety commonly ascribed to hypochondria, neurosis, or psychosomatic disorders. The range of known reaction to various sub-clinical deficiencies is a catalogue of contemporary complaint. It includes exhaustion, muscle ache and pain, nervousness, digestive upset, headache, fatigue, tingling, palpitations, poor concentration, and loss of appetite. After a lifetime of such metabolic injury, it can hardly be surprising that the body's principal organ systems should succumb to the ravages of heart attacks, circulatory disorders, cancer, diabetes, and other degenerative or metabolic diseases.

Biochemical Individuality and the Absurdity of "Average" Vitamin Requirements

Every individual has a set of vitamin needs as unique as his own fingerprints. Although no one would sensibly suggest that a lumberjack and a secretary consume the same number of calories, published nutritional tables often imply that everyone requires the same daily allowance of vitamins. The tyranny and absurdity of the "average" is obvious. While many of your vitamin requirements may approach a *normative* amount, the statistical probability is that your need for one or more of the vitamins is at dramatic odds with the "average." Because vitamins work together synergistically, or as a team, no metabolic process can operate with any more efficiency than that of its *least* effective component. If an individual wishes to manufacture wall clocks, he may find various suppliers who can provide him with as many as 20 timing mechanisms, 15 clock faces, and 9 cabinets per week. That he can produce no more than 9 finished timepieces in 7 days is readily apparent. In a similar manner, the productivity of your metabolic factories, or body cells, is determined and probably impaired by less-than-optimal intake of even a single vitamin.

Acquired Vitamin Dependence

When vitamin-depletion disease occurs, standard medical practice dictates that massive doses of the absent nutrient be administered over long periods of time. Once the victims of pellagra receive emergency treatment and are medically stabilized, they must consume approximately 600 mg, or 30 times the officially recommended daily allowance (U.S. RDA), of B_3, or niacin, per day for a number of years or their acute symptoms reappear. Similarly, the victims of pernicious anemia must ingest up to 400 mcg, or 65 times the standard U.S. RDA, of vitamin B_{12} to prevent recurrence of their disorder. Elderly patients, who often develop such signs of incipient scurvy as bleeding gums, spontaneous hemorrhages, and general malaise, must supplement their diets with more than 20 times the U.S. RDA of vitamin C before their symptoms cease. For unknown biochemical reasons, even temporary vitamin deprivation or depletion tends to elevate the body's needs for that vitamin on a more or less permanent basis.

Although you have probably never suffered from an overt vitamin-depletion disease, it is a virtual certainty that you have experienced some episodes of intense sub-clinical deficiency. The stresses of pregnancy, illness, tension, and anxiety all tend to increase your body's demand for vitamins. Periods of nutritional impoverishment typical of adolescence or economic hard times can reduce your vitamin intake. Such circumstances are common to all of us and create an abnormal, if temporary, gap between optimal vitamin intake and actual ingestion. They may trigger a permanent elevation in vitamin requirements. Given the possibility that many of us may suffer from long-term sub-clinical deficiencies, it is probable that greatly increased vitamin dosages are essential to correct injury done to deprived cells and tissues. To conclude that many of the common non-infectious illnesses develop because of an individual's far-from-average need for a particular vitamin or other nutrient is not unreasonable.

Vitamin Depletion Diseases: Ancient History or Modern Reality?

The recent government-financed Health and Nutrition Examination Studies (HANES) provide the nation with a first comprehensive evaluation of its dietary fitness. The results contradict the FDA's assumption that symptoms of clinical depletion diseases rarely occur in the United States and its conclusion that vitamins must, therefore, be amply supplied in the average American diet. Overt signs of actual or imminent depletion are widespread, though largely undetected. Adolescents, students, single people, chronic dieters, and the elderly, all of whom often achieve no more than a borderline nutritional status, are particularly vulnerable and frequently exhibit unmistakable symptoms of *nyctalopia,* or night blindness, scurvy, beri beri, and other depletion diseases. It is a current reality that more than 13 percent of "average"

Americans over 60 years of age have the serrations and fissures of the tongue symptomatic of incipient vitamin B₃ depletion, or pellagra. Similar numbers reveal the profound skeletal deterioration typical of vitamin D deficiencies leading to *osteoporosis* and *osteomalacia,* adult forms of rickets. Forty percent of the population, or close to 90 million people, show symptoms of visual deterioration typical of the vitamin A deficiency preceding night blindness. Although vitamin A is a fat-soluble vitamin normally stored in the liver and less vulnerable to depletion than water-soluble counterparts, an estimated 20 percent of all adults have the marginal vitamin A stores typical of the newborn, and another 10 percent have no vitamin A reserves at all. Because the dazzling effects of sunny beaches, winter snows, and overlit offices subtly deplete the body's stores of the vitamin, it is not surprising that two of five Americans from all socio-economic classes easily develop a potentially lethal depletion condition without knowing it. Although total blindness is the direct result of prolonged deficiency, inability to adapt to the glare of sunlight during the day or headlights at night contributes measurably to carnage on the nation's highways.

If the clinical symptoms of vitamin deficiency are as endemic as the HANES studies and subsequent surveys suggest, then it is reasonable to assume that large numbers of Americans suffer from sub-clinical deficiencies, while very few enjoy optimum vitamin intake. Because prolonged metabolic impairment undermines health and makes the body vulnerable to infectious diseases and degenerative disorders, vitamin supplementation seems advisable for most of us. Although many of the injurious effects of deprivation are irreversible, there is evidence that long-term saturation of long-deprived tissue with vitamins can arrest and to a degree correct cellular deterioration. Just as it would be unthinkable not to seek control over elevated blood sugar before the appearance of diabetes, it would be foolhardy not to attempt correction of sub-clinical vitamin deficiencies before the appearance of chronic or clinical deficiency symptoms. FDA Recommended Daily Allowances (U.S. RDAs), formulated to assure vitamin intake adequate for the prevention of overt disease, provide a safety factor intended to compensate for dietary vagaries, metabolic variation, and exceptional stress. These fail-safe margins cannot be expected to correct long-standing deficiencies. Because there has been a virtual moratorium on funding for vitamin research during recent decades, there has been little opportunity for the rigorous, controlled, and statistically significant testing of the effects that long-term, high-concentration vitamin supplementation has on human metabolism. While limited studies and the anecdotal reports of eminent vitamin-users are highly optimistic and suggestive, they do not constitute proof of efficacy. Evidence for the benefits of long-term, high-dosage vitamin supplementation currently comes from other sources.

Animal Breeders and Husbands: Evidence for the Benefits of Concentrated Vitamin Supplementation

Before a drug becomes available to humans, its effects on the metabolism of rats, white mice, or guinea pigs must be rigorously and extensively tested. Because of their evolutionary kinship with man, such laboratory animals provide a good, though imperfect, human proxy in the evaluation of substances intended for man's use. Over many years the results of animal studies have proved invaluable bellwethers of how human metabolism will respond not only to drugs but to industrial chemicals, food additives, insecticides, and related compounds as well. Although cattle, pigs, horses, and sheep share a similar evolutionary relationship to humans, their longer life spans and reproductive cycles, costly maintenance, and small number of offspring make them less suited to controlled laboratory experimentation than rodents. Nonetheless, domesticated animals have been the target of intensive scientific scrutiny for decades. Because of the enormous economic importance of attaining maximum growth with maximum efficiency in converting feed to flesh, most experimentation has focused on the nutritional biochemistry of livestock. As a result of tremendous research efforts, man probably knows more about the metabolism of his herd and racing animals than about his own nutritional chemistry. Since thoroughbred horses, pigs, sheep, cattle, and laboratory animals share a similar degree of biochemical affinity with man, it is curious that metabolic knowledge derived from animal husbandry is not more generally applied to humanity.

Farmers, justifiably interested in profit, feed their animals at "optimum" nutritional levels, while man is officially nourished at levels "adequate" to prevent disease. Animal breeders provide their herds with supplementary vitamins at concentrations not only sufficient to prevent deficiency disorders but at levels that assure maximum cell efficiency, growth, and good health. Such optimal vitamin concentrations are achieved when tissues are maintained at saturation levels throughout the life of the animal. Calves are fed for maximum rates of growth with vitamin A concentrations that are 20 to 25 times greater than the amounts necessary to prevent night blindness. Although overt clinical symptoms of pyridoxine, or vitamin B_6, depletion are not observed in growing piglets, biochemical evidence for sub-clinical B_6 deficiencies is often detected. A three- to fivefold increase in dietary levels of pyridoxine eliminates evidence of all biochemical disruptions and stimulates optimum growth. Similar results are obtained in chicks with B_6 supplementation in amounts 6 times that necessary to prevent clinical symptoms of depletion.

Although a pound-for-pound comparison of the vitamin needs for man and his domestic animals is obviously imperfect, it is significant that FDA Recommended Daily Allowances for humans fall far short of the U.S. Department of Agriculture recommendations for livestock and poultry. Vitamin A requirements on an equivalent weight basis are 150 percent greater for cattle, 200 percent greater for pigs, 250 percent greater for hens, and 500 percent greater for dogs. Recommendations for intake of B-complex vitamins and vitamin D reflect a comparable disparity. Among man's closest biochemical relatives are the apes, monkeys, and other primates. A weight-for-weight comparison reveals that their usual intake of ascorbic acid alone exceeds that of man by a factor of nearly 100.

Although the concept of optimal vitamin intake is well established for animals, the absence of relevant data does not allow the establishment of similar optimum levels for humans. All that is known for man are those concentrations of the various vitamins necessary to prevent clinical signs of deficiency or depletion. Because animals provide a reasonably reliable guide to human needs, there is merit in predicting that the benefits of improved health and performance, which accrue from saturating animal tissues with vitamins, might apply to human tissue as well. Extensive laboratory research is required to test the validity of such hypotheses. That medical and governmental authorities, committed to the principle of "adequate" rather than "optimal" nutrition, withhold funds for such experimentation is a cause for public concern. Culpability is compounded as the same authorities cite a "lack of evidence" for failing to underwrite the research necessary to obtain that very evidence, and lay the burden of proof on the shoulders of proponents clearly unable to finance such experimentation and study. Intransigence in the face of declining life expectancy and general health seems misguided. It has its repercussions as Americans increasingly mistrust the motivation and capacity of their government, medical institutions, and physicians to resolve contemporary health problems.

Simply living longer is no longer the American dream. It is the quality of life, not its length, that is now of prime importance. Modern medicine, with all its technical virtuosity, appears impotent against the degenerative diseases that increasingly undermine the young, condemn the mature, and make the aged body a prison. While viewing extraordinary medical feats that maintain life against all odds with detached awe, the public clearly excels its traditional health-care custodians in recognizing that an ounce of preventive medicine is worth a pound of curative technique. That established authorities are not more effective in controlling the quality of the food and environment, so intimately associated with life expectancy and good health, is a source of disillusionment. Given their apparent wrongheadedness, the individual must take growing responsibility for the protection and maintenance of his own health. Intelligent self-preservation requires close attention to personal lifestyle and eating habits.

Because they are foods essential to cellular and tissue metabolism, your wise use of vitamins and vitamin supplements must be in the interests of improved nutrition. That the vitamin-impoverished American diet generally requires supplementation to meet official Recommended Daily Allowances is probable. Whether your choice of such supplementation can compensate for years of subclinical deficiencies is another question. The judicious addition of vitamins to your diet at higher concentrations will probably not cure diseases. It may help prevent them.

3

Your Vitamin Needs: An Establishment Viewpoint

Dine on little. Sup on less.

— CERVANTES

WHAT ARE *YOUR* REQUIREMENTS?

There is no easy or absolute answer to this question. Until nutrition becomes an exact science, the issue of vitamin needs will continue to attract controversy as moths to a flame. Although no one denies that vitamins are necessary for life, there is little consensus about which vitamins are essential, what quantities are desirable, and how they should be supplied. Whenever any standards or guidelines for vitamin intake are offered, the propositions and their proponents become the target of passionate criticism, exaggeration, distortion, scorn, and abuse. Business enterprises, the press, and "concerned" citizens often seize such proposals for the purposes of enhancing profit, creating sensational news stories, or grinding personal axes to a fine and combative edge. Government agencies and medical cartels share similar propensities for misrepresentation and vitriol as they wage campaigns that portray dissenters from nutritional orthodoxy as freaks, faddists, and subversives. The vitamin battlefield is metaphorically bloody. Where does such partisan fury leave you, whose only stake in the controversy is the quality of your life and health? Can you glean nutritional truths about your vitamin needs amidst such tirade and tempest? It is not easy. It is worth a try.

THE FOOD AND NUTRITION BOARD OF THE NATIONAL RESEARCH COUNCIL: RECOMMENDED DIETARY ALLOWANCES (RDAs)

The National Academy of Sciences is America's most powerful and prestigious scientific organization. It unites the nation's foremost physicists, chemists, biologists, and physicians into a forum for integrating, evaluating, and directing scientific and medical endeavors. Its Food and Nutrition Board is charged with periodically assessing the nation's diet. Members regularly meet to review and revise published recommendations concerning the numbers and quantities of nutrients thought advisable for good nutrition. Its findings represent reasoned opinion rather than scientific certainty and are prone to frequent modification in light of new scientific and medical evidence. While not legally binding on regulatory agencies within the government, its recommendations weigh heavily on the policy-making scales that control and direct American agriculture and health-care practices. Because of its preeminent position, the Board is frequently abused as a self-serving Polonius, protecting the nutritional status quo, or exalted as an enlightened Prometheus, dispensing absolute nutritional truths. Neither portrayal is fair. The eighth edition of its *Recommended Dietary Allowances,* published in 1974, is a moderate document that reflects a reasoned consensus of opinion among a group of rational scientific thinkers. They profess no ultimate dietary wisdom, admit their uncertainties about many questions, and confess that establishing nutritional recommendations is not unlike working a jigsaw puzzle with many of the pieces missing.

Current Food and Nutrition Board thought about the dietary need for protein, twelve vitamins, and six minerals (RDAs) is summarized by the chart on pages 64–65. Although the importance of certain fatty acids, carbohydrates, water, and choline is recognized, fixed recommendations for these substances are not provided. Two B-complex vitamins—biotin and pantothenic acid—and nine minerals are similarly identified as necessary, but currently lack RDAs for want of sufficient data. (Estimated ranges for their safe and adequate daily intake are listed in Appendix D, page 234.)

In defining the philosophy that governed the formulation of its recommendations, the 1974 Board adhered to the principle that health is a state of physical, mental, and social well-being, not merely the absence of disease or infirmity. In putting theory to practice, it expressed many concerns, caveats, and reservations about its own methodology and recommendations.

- The 1974 Board recognizes that present nutritional knowledge is incomplete, and that man's requirements for many nutrients have not been established. For these reasons it recommends that you consume as varied a selection of foods as is practicable, acceptable, and palatable.

- The Board expresses considerable concern about the absolute certainty of the nutritional evidence at its disposal. Although information from human research is obviously most desirable and weighs most heavily in its decision-making processes, much of the precision, accuracy, and applicability of the available data is questionable. Because investigations of man involve great cost, ethical prohibitions, social taboos, and long periods of time, many recommendations are necessarily based on the results of a limited number of studies with a limited number of subjects. Judgements must fall back on human analogies drawn from animal studies, food assays, and less-than-per-

Adapted from Recommended Daily
of the Food and Nutrition Board, National

Age (years)	Weight (lbs)	Height (in)	Protein (g)	Fat-Soluble Vitamins[b]			Water-Soluble Vitamins[b]	
				Vitamin A (IU)	Vitamin D (IU)	Vitamin E (IU)	Ascorbic Acid C (mg)	Folic Acid — (mcg)
Infants								
0.0–0.5	13	24	1/lb.	1,400	400	4.5	35	30
0.5–1.0	20	28	0.9/lb.	2,000	400	6	35	45
Children								
1–3	29	35	23	2,000	400	7.5	45	100
4–6	44	44	30	2,500	400	9	45	200
7–10	62	52	34	3,500	400	10.5	45	300
Males								
11–14	99	62	45	5,000	400	12	50	400
15–18	145	69	56	5,000	400	15	60	400
19–22	154	70	56	5,000	300	15	60	400
23–50	154	70	56	5,000	200	15	60	400
51+	154	70	56	5,000	200	15	60	400
Females								
11–14	101	62	46	4,000	400	12	50	400
15–18	120	64	46	4,000	400	12	60	400
19–22	120	64	44	4,000	300	12	60	400
23–50	120	64	44	4,000	200	12	60	400
51+	120	64	44	4,000	200	12	60	400
Pregnant			+30	5,000	+200	+3	+20	+400
Lactating			+20	6,000	+200	+4.5	+40	+100

[a]The allowances are intended to provide for individual variations among most normal persons as they live in the United States under usual environmental stresses. Diets should be based on a variety of common foods in order to provide other nutrients for which human requirements have been less well defined.

[b]IU = international units; mg = milligrams; mcg = μg = micrograms. The 1980 edition of *Recommended Dietary Allowances* expresses the figures for the fat-soluble vitamins as mg of retinol equivalents (vit. A), mg of cholecalciferol (vit. D), and mg of alpha-tocopherol equivalents (vit. E). Since supplement labels express these values in IUs, rough equivalents have been provided in IUs for each.

fect dietary surveys among apparently healthy people. In the absence of scientifically rigorous data it is not surprising that Board members are not always in agreement about what concentrations of a nutrient genuinely fulfill various requirements. In suggesting some allowances that do no more than prevent clinical symptoms of deficiency, they recognize that such

Dietary Allowances (RDAs, as revised, 1980)[a]
Academy of Sciences–National Research Council

| Water-Soluble Vitamins cont'd[b] | | | | | | | Minerals[b] | | | | | |
Thiamin B$_1$ (mg)	Riboflavin B$_2$ (mg)	Niacin B$_3$ (mg)	Vitamin B$_6$ (mg)	Vitamin B$_{12}$ (mcg)	Biotin[c] (mcg)	Pantothenic Acid[c] (mg)	Calcium (mg)	Phosphorus (mg)	Iodine (mg)	Iron (mg)	Magnesium (mg)	Zinc (mg)
0.3	0.4	6	0.3	0.5	35	2	360	240	.04	10	50	3
0.5	0.6	8	0.6	1.5	50	3	540	360	.05	15	70	5
0.7	0.8	9	0.9	2.0	65	3	800	800	.07	15	150	10
0.9	1.0	11	1.3	2.5	85	3–4	800	800	.09	10	200	10
1.2	1.4	16	1.6	3.0	120	4–5	800	800	.12	10	250	10
1.4	1.6	18	1.8	3.0	100–200	4–7	1,200	1,200	.15	18	350	15
1.4	1.7	18	2.0	3.0	100–200	4–7	1,200	1,200	.15	18	400	15
1.5	1.7	19	2.2	3.0	100–200	4–7	800	800	.15	10	350	15
1.4	1.6	18	2.2	3.0	100–200	4–7	800	800	.15	10	350	15
1.2	1.4	16	2.2	3.0	100–200	4–7	800	800	.15	10	350	15
1.1	1.3	15	1.8	3.0	100–200	4–7	1,200	1,200	.15	18	300	15
1.1	1.3	14	2.0	3.0	100–200	4–7	1,200	1,200	.15	18	300	15
1.1	1.3	14	2.0	3.0	100–200	4–7	800	800	.15	18	300	15
1.0	1.2	13	2.0	3.0	100–200	4–7	800	800	.15	18	300	15
1.0	1.2	13	2.0	3.0	100–200	4–7	800	800	.15	10	300	15
+0.4	+0.3	+2	+0.6	+1.0			+400	+400	+.025	[d]	450	20
+0.5	+0.5	+5	+0.5	+1.0			+400	+400	+.05	[d]	450	25

[c]The figures for biotin and pantothenic acid are from the 1980 *Recommended Dietary Allowances'* table of "Estimated Safe and Adequate Daily Dietary Intakes of Selected Vitamins and Minerals." The Board gives these figures in a separate table "because there is less information on which to base allowances."

[d]This increased requirement cannot be met by ordinary diets; therefore, the use of 30–60 mg of supplemental iron is recommended during pregnancy and for 2–3 months afterward.

amounts do not maintain maximum tissue stores and may fall short of optimum concentrations.

● Although the Board emphasizes its ignorance of any convincing evidence of unique benefits derived from the ingestion of a large excess of any one nutrient, e.g. a vitamin, it does not discount the potential advantages of moderate surplus intake.[1] *Its far greater concern is with the cumulative effects of even small vitamin deficits, which may lead to deficiencies.* Because the human body is so biochemically flexible, it may successfully cope with temporary deprivations. Such short-term adaptation may ultimately undermine good health in the face of prolonged deficiencies.

● Because its recommendations are concerned with daily food allowances and are not related to the quality of national, regional, or local food supplies, individual dietary planning must compensate for predictable losses of nutrients, e.g. vitamins and minerals, resulting from transportation, storage, processing, and preparation.

● The individual is urged to realize that his nutritional requirements may vary from the average and from time to time in his life. Among healthy individuals this variability involves age, sex, body size, genetic makeup, medical history, and the quality of the physical and psychological environment. Although the Board feels that its recommended allowances tend to provide protective margins, unique factors such as infections, metabolic disorders, chronic diseases, and drugs may render RDAs inadequate for many individuals.

● The 1974 *Recommended Dietary Allowances* takes elaborate pains to dispel the myth of the "average" man and to define the legitimate use of RDAs. It makes clear that recommended allowances can only be meaningful within the framework of statistical probability and cannot predict nutritional adequacy for any individual. In a similar fashion, general statements to the effect that "Vitamins and minerals are abundant in the food we eat; therefore, there is no problem of nutritional deficiency" are invalid. The

---

1. Except for calorie rich foods that may lead to obesity, or vitamins A and D and some minerals, which may prove toxic in large quantities.

supposed justification for such statements relies on the *range* of individual needs and nutritional intake. In any population numbers of people with low requirements and high intake for a nutrient are statistically balanced by numbers of people who have high requirements but low intake for the same nutrient. The average between the two groups does not identify those with dietary insufficiency, let alone reveal that any inadequacy exists at all. In accepting the results of the Ten-State Nutritional Survey (HEW, 1972), the Board has identified the fallacy of averages, as this screening clearly reveals that "even in a country as well supplied with nutrients as the U.S., a portion of the population obviously has a less than adequate diet."

The scientific wisdom, balance, and moderation of the 1974 Food and Nutrition Board's RDAs may be admired. Their abuse by the FDA may be abhorred.

THE FOOD AND DRUG ADMINISTRATION: U.S. RECOMMENDED DAILY ALLOWANCES (U.S. RDAs)

The FDA is the government agency responsible for protecting your health by regulating the quality and availability of the medicines and foodstuffs you can obtain in the marketplace. Its task is awesome—one made infinitely complex in recent years by the proliferation of novel drugs and food products resulting from spectacular advances in technological chemistry. The FDA commissioner annually receives thousands of applications for the testing and evaluation of new substances. The demand for speedy approval is immense. Pharmaceutical houses, food processors, and manufacturers of agricultural compounds all exert tremendous and subtle pressure in their quest for FDA permission to market new products. They are joined by consumer and public interest groups who often complain that archaic testing procedures and rigid bureaucratic attitudes prevent Americans from speedily enjoying the fruits of modern research. The dilemma is clear. If antibiotics had been subjected to the most scientifically rigorous, hence ideal, testing techniques, penicillin would have just recently achieved widespread availability, and tetracycline might still be prohibited except for limited use among carefully controlled numbers of people. Although the withholding of such substances seems unthinkable today, the caution that restricted availability of thalidomide in the early 1960s undoubtedly prevented the birth of many cruelly deformed American children. You might wish that similar caution had been exerted over the release of liquid protein diets for weight reduction.

In 1963, apparently reacting with alarm to the increasing number of vitamin and mineral food supplements available to the public, the FDA began to hear evidence for the purposes of defining appropriate formulation and labeling regulations for such products. Although no one contests the legitimacy of such FDA interest, the agency's inept handling of its inquiry and the draconian nature of its proposed regulations compromised confidence in its capacity to function impartially in the interests of your health.

Interpreting the public's burgeoning interest in vitamin and mineral supplements as tangible evidence of a growing disaffection with traditional health-care authority, the agency and its spokesmen attempted to quash this heresy by virtually regulating such products out of existence. Instead of quelling a rebellion the FDA, and to a lesser extent its food industry and medical establishment allies, reaped a whirlwind of public, scientific, judicial, Congressional, and Presidential criticism, wrath, and ultimate censure. It is a sorry tale.

The commissioner's initial proposals appeared in the *Federal Register* of June 20, 1962. They bore the unmistakable hallmark of the paternalism and condescension that the alliance of government and medicine had long used to cow the public into uncritical submission. In essence, they implied that the average consumer is a nutritional idiot unaware of his vitamin needs and is easy prey for scare tactics concerning an "improbable" lack of vitamins in his diet and the ill health that might result from such inadequacy. To protect the "common" man from his own ignorance, the FDA sought to limit the nutrient content and labeling of all supplements to eight vitamins (A; B_1, or thiamin; B_2, or riboflavin; B_3, or niacin; B_6; B_{12}; C; and D) and four minerals (iron, phosphorus, calcium, and iodine) recognized as essential by the Food and Nutrition Board. Other known and necessary vitamins and minerals were regarded as so plentiful in the diet that, while they might be included in a supplement, they could not be listed on the label since such identification might imply a "false" value for the consumer. A further proposal intended to supplant identifications of Minimum Daily Requirements (MDRs)[2] with Recommended *Daily* Allowances (U.S. RDAs) derived from the Food and Nutrition Board's similar Recommended *Dietary* Allowances (RDAs), along with stated maximum and minimum dosages. The latter regulation was defended as necessary to prevent the inclusion of excessive vitamin and mineral quantities in a supplement as a gimmick to separate the gullible from their gold.

Reaction to the commissioner's proposals was unequivocal. Having invited comment about the tentative rules and regulations, the FDA was deluged by an unprecedented wave of criticism that united bricklayers with Nobel Prize winners. With their nutritional freedom of choice in jeopardy, a once-docile populace responded to the threat of further bureaucratic control over their lives in no uncertain terms. Daunted by the depth, extent, and prestige of negative critical response, the agency withdrew its proposals.

After a four-year "cooling off" period the FDA resumed its militant offensive against nutritional heresy by

2. MDRs were initially established in 1941 and were designed to protect soldiers and civilians from vitamin depletion as the nation was about to go to war. Re-evaluations of MDR values by 1963 were logical in light of advances in knowledge of human nutrition and metabolism that had taken place during the preceding twenty years.

publishing a revision of its tentative rules and regulations. Although there is little concrete evidence that either agribusiness or the medical establishment exerted coercive pressure on the agency, the new proposals might well have been penned in medical association or food industry boardrooms. Not only were U.S. RDAs to replace traditional MDRs, but any supplement containing more than 150 percent of the Recommended Daily Allowance of a nutrient was to be considered a drug and could only be obtained with a physician's prescription. To retain its classification as a food supplement, no product could contain nutrient concentrations greater than the amounts stipulated by the U.S. RDAs. Formulations with vitamin and mineral levels falling between 100 and 150 percent of the U.S. RDAs were eventually to be ranked as non-prescription, or over-the-counter, medications.

In seeking to eliminate products that were perceived as irrational, the new regulations not only sought to control ingredient concentrations, but attempted to dictate which combinations of vitamins and minerals could be included in a single supplement. To further restrict the manufacturer, product labels could not suggest that foods might be nutritionally deficient because of soil depletion or harvesting, storage, processing, and/or food preparation losses. Claims that ingredients were derived from natural rather than synthetic sources or that vitamins might prevent or cure disease—even those resulting from nutritional deficiencies—were to be disallowed. Not only were manufacturers to be enjoined from any labeling statement that suggested *any* use or function for their product, they were to substitute the following warning in place of any promotional claims:

Vitamins and minerals are supplied in abundant amounts in the foods we eat. The Food and Nutrition Board of the National Research Council recommends that dietary needs be satisfied by foods. Except for persons with special medical needs, there is no scientific basis for recommending routine use of dietary supplements.

If such autocratic proposals were intended as an opiate for the restive and questioning masses, the pontifical language of their formulation and the authoritarian method of their presentation failed to provide an antidote to dissent. The new rules and regulations instead stirred angry criticism from layman and scientist alike. Consumers, weary of having their lives programmed by big business interests and government bureaucracy, carried their protests to Congress. They were joined by prominent scientists, who were outraged by the FDA's flagrant abuse of recognized scientific principle, evidence, and practice. Among the first to decry the FDA proposals were members of the Food and Nutrition Board, who objected to having their avowed value judgements taken out of proper context and restated as absolute nutritional gospel. Comprehensive dietary surveys and evaluations of national eating patterns—initiated in response to FDA assertions—challenged *a priori* assumptions that common foods are richly endowed with either vitamins or minerals and demonstrated that inadequate nutrition is typical of significant numbers of Americans from all socio-economic classes. Even physicians and nutritionists were critical of the absolutist assertion that there is no scientific basis for regular dietary supplementation. It is established practice to advise the addition of vitamins to the diet of any normal infant, child, or adolescent. The same is true for any otherwise healthy adult if his eating habits are at all irregular, prohibit the intake of certain foods, or for any reason threaten the adequacy of his vitamin supply. Such broad-spectrum rejection of the FDA's position reflected profound concern that when a federal agency begins to dictate what is *scientifically true* and *accurate,* it is clearly later than anyone thinks.

With its attempted imposition of repressive controls over vitamin and mineral products, the FDA inadvertently exposed itself to intense public scrutiny, stimulated broad inquiry into the nation's nutritional well-being, and renewed debate about the relative merits of food supplementation. The controversy, which has continued since 1966, has resulted in a severe condemnation of the agency's attitudes, and limited its powers to regulate and control the composition of vitamin and mineral products. During these intervening years there has been little willing modification of its implacable stance, and its categorical public pronouncements have continued to make it an unenviable target for criticism—some of it appropriate, some of it extreme. Among the many allegations of agency partisanship and lack of objectivity are a number that deserve review. They include charges that the FDA is guilty of—

- *exaggerating public fears concerning hypervitaminosis, or vitamin "overdose."* According to most recent medical evidence, hypervitaminosis resulting from the intake of water-soluble vitamins is a biochemical impossibility. Amounts exceeding tissue-saturation levels are apparently excreted from the body with no ill effect to tissue or metabolism. Although fat-soluble A, D, and E may be stored in the liver and other tissues, it takes massive and repeated doses to produce even mild toxicity. For example, the adult liver alone can absorb up to 500,000 International Units (IU) of vitamin A with little or no ill effect. Only a single dose of 2,000,000 IU or prolonged ingestion of over 100,000 IU per day will predictably produce symptoms of tissue overloading. Since 2 ounces of ordinary beef liver contain at least 30,000 IU of vitamin A, attempts to classify supplements containing more than 7,500 IU as drugs seem patently absurd. According to FDA reasoning you would need a physician's prescription to purchase a lamb chop, a sweet potato, or most organ meats. Even the so-called "mega" dose regimens typically call for no more than 25,000 IU of the vitamin per day.

Although vitamin E toxicity is virtually unknown, vitamin D poisoning is possible, but only in extravagant doses—10 to 20 times the U.S. RDA for the vitamin. Symptoms of hypervitaminosis disap-

pear on cessation of intake and produce no known
bodily damage. You may well wonder at FDA attempts to control vitamin availability, when the
ubiquitous aspirin causes one American death every
three days. No one has ever died from an overdose
of vitamins.

- *intentionally confusing vitamins with drugs.* It is unfortunate that most vitamin supplements are compounded in tablet, drop, or capsule form and are
ordinarily sold in pharmacies rather than supermarkets. Vitamins are just as much foods as are carbohydrates, proteins, and fats. Unlike drugs, they are essential to life, become an integral part of all body
cells, and are metabolized in much the same way as
other food elements. They produce their effects in
cooperation with one another and as natural components of the enzymes, which regulate normal biochemical processes. In excess they are excreted or
stored without interfering in normal body functioning. Drugs are substances typically alien to body
chemistry, work independently, are apt to disrupt
normal biochemical pathways, and tend to produce
severe side effects, even death, in excess.

    By attempting to classify vitamins as drugs in
concentrations exceeding 150 percent of U.S. RDA
values, the FDA appeals to justifiable public caution
about consuming any substance presumed to be a
medication because of its pill, capsule, or tablet formulation. This misrepresentation may serve FDA
purposes but does violence to fundamental biochemical truths and constitutes an insult to the public
intelligence.

- *intentionally misinterpreting Food and Nutrition
Board RDAs.* In its adaptation of values established
by the Board, the FDA eliminated the members'
carefully expressed caveats, cautions, and concerns
about their findings. By widely publicizing reasoned
opinion as if it were nutritional truth, the agency
does harm to respected scientific principle and sullies

the reputation of those whose authority it invokes.[3] By attempting to convert fluctuating estimates of nutritional needs (RDAs) to absolute and inviolable numbers (U.S. RDAs), the agency imposes arbitrary limits on the formulation of vitamin supplements and exerts subtle suasion over the minds of a trusting public. That the same public is led to confuse individual needs with some mythical average is appalling.

Equally distressing is the possibility (as some Congressmen have charged) that U.S. RDA levels are kept purposefully low because of agribusiness lobbying and pressure. That the food industry benefits from minimum rather than maximum recommended allowances is undeniable. Lower U.S. RDA values make company products appear nutritionally richer. Prime examples are breakfast cereals that may now boast 100 percent U.S. RDAs for most vitamins while being nutritionally inferior to the fruit and milk customarily added to make them palatable.

● *arbitrarily establishing fixed and rigid formulas for supplements.* An initial FDA attempt to dictate what vitamins and what minerals might be included in a supplement has been struck down by Congress and the President. In its zeal to prevent irresponsible manufacturers from fabricating and marketing irrational combinations of vitamins and minerals, the agency sought to limit products to five basic preparations: a) all the vitamins and all the minerals; b) all the vitamins alone; c) all the minerals alone; d) all the vitamins with a supplement of iron; or e) any single vitamin *or* mineral. In seeking to define such allowable combinations, the tentative regulations denied nutrient couplings that frequently occur in Nature, e.g. bioflavonoids and vitamin C. Such restrictions

3. You may wonder at FDA attempts to identify its own positions with the prestige of the National Academy of Sciences as it creates inevitable confusion by calling its dietary proposals Recommended *Daily* Allowances (U.S. RDAs) in obvious imitation of the Food and Nutrition Board's Recommended *Dietary* Allowances (RDAs).

are not too far removed from dictating your daily menu, e.g. allowing you a steak and baked potato for dinner while forbidding you a salad.

● *diverting proper investigative attention from more critical issues.* If the FDA had exhibited equivalent ardor in controlling and regulating the pesticides, food additives, and carcinogens that pollute food and demonstrably lead to human illness, its war against vitamins might have attained greater credibility and stature. In choosing to spend more than fifteen years and millions of dollars in attempting to regulate a simple therapy involving virtually no risk to humans, the FDA may be justifiably accused of misplacing its priorities. The importance of vitamins in man's diet has long been recognized. The need for butylated hydroxytoluene (BHT), nitrosamines, red dye #3, and polychlorobiphenyls (PCBs) in human nutrition has not been established.

● *initiating or perpetuating nutritional myths.* Among various fallacies the FDA has actively promulgated, tacitly supported, or failed to challenge are a number with broad implications for national and personal health. They have included implied or stated arguments that—

● ● *inadequate nutrition is virtually nonexistent in the United States.* Recent dietary surveys suggest that more than one third of the population consumes less than U.S. RDAs for vitamin A. Medical journals and health agencies increasingly assail the nutritional status of the average American, citing wide gaps between nutritional needs and supplies, resulting from poor eating habits, fad diets, drugs, and the consumption of heavily processed foods. Indeed, a 1980 report from the U.S. Department of Agriculture warns that most women between 23 and 50 consume only 1,500 food calories a day— 500 calories short of the Recommended Daily Dietary Allowance for this age group. According to

Department nutritionists, it is virtually impossible to design such a low-calorie diet, i.e. 1,500 daily calories or less, that meets even U.S. RDA recommendations for all vitamins and minerals—without supplementation.

• • *individual nutritional needs can be predicted from statistical averages and that adherence to U.S. RDAs should fulfill your nutritional requirements.* Sophisticated tools for precise nutritional analyses are currently lacking, e.g. mass-screening programs for detecting individual malnutrition (similar to those used to uncover cancer or tuberculosis). Vitamin assay techniques, essential for accurately measuring nutrient concentrations in various body tissues and fluids, are now too primitive and too costly to be used in determining nutritional well-being.

The range of human requirements, as opposed to allowances, for various nutrients has been established for fewer than a dozen substances. Where known, there is typically a two- to tenfold variation in need and demand from individual to individual. Just as it would be ludicrous to give every diabetic the same dose of insulin, it would be foolish to expect that standardized U.S. RDAs can fulfill the requirements of 95 to 99 percent of the population (as the FDA claims). Such recommended allowances are essentially derived from research intended to determine minimum needs to avoid disease. Their use in determining optimal personal vitamin intake cannot be scientifically justified.

• • *if a vitamin lacks a fixed U.S. RDA or if a specific need in human nutrition has not been established, it is best to discount the nutrient.* The Food and Nutrition Board candidly admits difficulty in establishing Recommended Dietary Allowances for various vitamins. As a result, a B-complex vitamin like *pantothenic acid* currently lacks an RDA. The fact that it is required in human nutrition is unquestioned.

Other nutrients, such as *choline* and *biotin,* are required by the body but may be provided by intestinal bacteria, and individuals may or may not require extrinsic dietary sources of supply depending on their unique biochemical demands. That *tocopherol,* or vitamin E, and *pyridoxine,* or B_6, were not officially recognized as vitamins until 1968 indicates that the metabolic function of various dietary substances is not easily determined and that the discovery of additional and essential vitamins may be predicted.

THE COURTS, THE CONGRESS, AND THE PRESIDENT: YOUR NUTRITIONAL FREEDOM OF CHOICE

In January of 1973 the FDA commissioner announced his intention of instituting final rules and regulations for vitamin supplements that included most of the foregoing scientifically questionable stipulations and interpretations. Although the new proposals were intended to take effect the following summer, implementation was enjoined by judicial decree. An Appeals Court action of August 1974 invalidated the FDA provision that would have classified any supplement with more than 150 percent of a U.S. RDA as a drug. The decision also allowed a greater number of ingredient combinations than approved by the agency and further delayed institution of the new rules and regulations.

After considerable investigation and debate, Congress enacted a Freedom of Nutrition bill that was signed into law by President Ford in the spring of 1976. The bill specifically forbids the FDA to establish maximum limits on the potency of any vitamin or mineral, or to restrict the combination or numbers of any vitamin, mineral, or other ingredient in a food supplement intended for use by adults or children over 12 years of age. Furthermore, such pro-

U.S. Recommended Daily Allowances

	Fat-Soluble Vitamins[a]			Water-Soluble Vitamins[a]			
	Vitamin A (IU)	Vitamin D (IU)	Vitamin E (IU)	Vitamin C (mg)	Folic Acid — (mcg)	Thiamin B₁ (mg)	Riboflavin B₂ (mg)
Infants							
Lower limit	1,250	200	5	20	100	.35	.4
U.S. RDA	1,500	400	5	35	100	.5	.6
Upper limit	1,500	400	5	35	100	.5	.6
Children under 4 years of age							
Lower limit	1,250	200	5	20	100	.35	.4
U.S. RDA	2,500	400	10	40	200	.7	.8
Upper limit	2,500	400	15	60	300	1.05	1.2
Adults and children 4 or more years of age							
Lower limit	2,500	200	15	30	200	.75	.8
U.S. RDA	5,000	400	30	60	400	1.5	1.7
Pregnant or lactating women							
Lower limit	5,000	400	30	60	400	1.5	1.7
U.S. RDA	8,000	400	30	60	800	1.7	2
Upper limit	8,000	400	60	120	800	3	3.4

[a]IU = international units; mg = milligrams; mcg = μg = micrograms.

ducts cannot be compositionally limited by attempting to classify them as prescription drugs. Such judicial, legislative, and presidential contravention of FDA intent and authority was without precedent. It left the agency with few responsibilities for nutritional supplement products beyond ensuring their purity, safety, guaranteed minimum potency, and labeling accuracy.

Following this stunning vote of "no confidence," the FDA commissioner invoked his restricted mandate and in October 1976 issued final regulations governing vitamin and mineral products. The new provisions apply to supplements entering the marketplace after January 1, 1978. They are principally concerned with products intended for

(U.S. RDAs) for Vitamins and Minerals

| Water-Soluble Vitamins cont'd[a] | | | | | Minerals[a] | | | | | | |
Niacin B₃ (mg)	Vitamin B₆ (mg)	Vitamin B₁₂ (mcg)	Biotin — (mcg)	Pantothenic Acid — (mg)	Calcium (mg)	Phosphorus (mg)	Iodine (mg)	Iron (mg)	Magnesium (mg)	Copper (mg)	Zinc (mg)
4.5	.35	1.5	50	2.5	125	125	.035	5	40	.5	4
8	.4	2	50	3	600	500	.045	15	70	.6	5
8	.4	2	50	3	600	500	.045	15	70	.6	5
4.5	.35	1.5	75	2.5	125	125	.035	5	40	.5	4
9	.7	3	150	5	800	800	.07	10	200	1	8
13.5	1.05	4.5	225	7.5	1,200	1,200	.105	15	300	1.5	12
10	1	3	150	5	125	125	.075	9	100	1	7.5
20	2	6	300	10	1,000	1,000	.15	18	400	2	15
20	2	6	300	10	125	125[b]	.15	18	100	1	7.5
20	2.5	8	300	10	1,300	1,300[b]	.15	18	450	2	15
40	4	12	600	20	2,000	2,000[b]	.3	60	800	4	30

[b]Optional for pregnant or lactating women. When present, the quantity of phosphorus may not be greater than the quantity of calcium.

use by pregnant or nursing (lactating) women, infants, and children under 4 years of age. In the name of safety these supplements must adhere to specific quantitative and qualitative formulations.

Labels for all supplements are now to list their product contents in terms of International Units (IU) of activity for vitamins A, D, and E, and units of weight (grams, milligrams, or micrograms) for all other vitamins and minerals. Labels must also provide conversions of these units into percentages of U.S. Adult RDAs. If any food or supplement product contains more than 2 percent of any U.S. RDA for a particular nutrient, that percentage must be identified.

INTERPRETATION OF THE U.S. RDAs

Current FDA recommended daily allowances are on pages 78–79. Although unreliable predictors of your personal vitamin needs, they may be used as minimal guidelines for ensuring probable freedom from depletion disorders. By taking advantage of the new labeling laws that went into effect on July 1, 1978, for canned, boxed, bottled, and frozen foods, you may estimate how effectively your diet fulfills these reactionary FDA recommendations. Keep a record of the food you consume for a period of from three to five days—specifically noting the percentage concentrations of each vitamin listed on the nutritional information panels of your food choices. Intake for *each* of the three fat-soluble and nine water-soluble vitamins should total 100 percent of its appropriate U.S. RDA for every day of your survey. If your normal diet fails to meet these minimal concentrations—*which is quite likely* —you have probably been experiencing prolonged nutritional deficiencies that have consistently but subtly undermined your health and well-being.

Because the disparity between your usual intake and FDA recommendations is apt to be shocking, increasing your consumption to meet U.S. RDA standards will predictably demand dramatic alteration in your diet—*often introducing undesirable calories and requiring the use of a single or multiple vitamin supplement*—to meet all prescribed standards. However, limiting your consumption to such officially sanctioned and conservative quotas can do predictably little to correct the injuries of past vitamin deprivation. Such half measures almost certainly will not meet your ideal metabolic requirements, which depend on such individual variables as your unique biochemical heritage, age, sex, eating habits, medical and nutritional history, lifestyle, and the environment in which you live. That those quantities essential for the most effective bodily function greatly exceed U.S. RDA recommendations for most of us is probable. That the FDA—the legal custodian and "scientific" watchdog of our food supply—has attempted to impose "adequate" rather than "optimal" vitamin nutrition on most Americans is a certainty.

AN AFTERWORD

It is unfortunate that so potentially valuable a personal and public ally as the FDA has exposed itself to loss of public esteem in its curious attack on vitamin and mineral supplements. Many of its intentions were well and logically conceived. Their intrinsic value was unfortunately undermined as agency positions hardened and official language became increasingly inflexible.

Vitamins and minerals, like all substances in the marketplace including more traditional foods, are subject to abuse. There are certainly unscrupulous vitamin salesmen and manufacturers just as there are unscrupulous doctors, lawyers, and priests. To assume that all are charlatans, quacks, or hucksters is patently unreasonable, as is the tacit belief that the consumer is a hapless dolt, incapable of making intelligent nutritional judgements and choices.

4

Vitamin Profiles

*Facts are the bricks and reason the mortar of
good judgement.*

— EMERY

In her creation of vitamin and vitaminlike compounds
Nature showed scant regard for man's compulsion to reduce her mysteries to precise verbal descriptions and formulations. Their universal distribution among all living
creatures, their biochemical versatility, and their chame-
leon-like resemblance to other metabolic molecules defy
attempts by biochemists, physicians, and wordsmiths to
capture the qualities of vitamins in any single, compact,
and exclusive word-portrait.

Although a consensual definition is lacking, vitamins
do share a number of characteristics about which there is
little disagreement. Like proteins, carbohydrates, and fats,
they are organic molecules composed of carbon, hydrogen, and oxygen. Unlike inorganic minerals, vitamins
must be manufactured from raw food materials by living
organisms, but like their mineral counterparts are essential for *all* life[1] in minute quantities. Some function as

---

1. It is a wonder of Nature and major evidence for the Theory of
Evolution that all organisms—ranging from microbes to man—require most
of the same vitamin or vitamin-like molecules for life. Only vitamin B_{12},
unneeded by plant cells, is in the exclusive domain of animal metabolism.

co-enzymes critical to the growth, maintenance, and repair of every living cell. Others, also co-enzymes, control biochemical processes among specialized cells whose chemical products coordinate and unify the billions of cells and numerous tissues comprising any complex organism. The absence or depletion of even a single vitamin causes biochemical disruption—whether in an alga, amoeba, aster, eagle, elephant, or man—that produces ill health, and eventually leads to a specific disease condition, even death.

VITAMINS AND HORMONES

Although the foregoing may pinpoint many of the essential qualities of vitamins, it fails to distinguish such substances from hormones, which are also organic molecules synthesized by living organisms and utilized in small amounts for the regulation of tissues and cells. Arbitrary and manmade distinctions between the two classes of compound often stipulate that "hormones" must be synthesized by the organism that employs them, while "vitamins" cannot be manufactured by the user and must be supplied from outside sources. Thus, the ascorbic acid created according to genetic instructions in the cells of a rat must be considered a hormone in that animal but a vitamin (C) in man and apes, who lack the necessary genetic machinery for such synthesis.

Vitamin Sources and Supplies: Fragile and Unreliable

Whether human vitamins can be defined in terms of their exclusive need to be supplied from your diet is debatable. The distinction certainly fails when accepting the traditional notion that a morsel in the mouth automatically becomes fuel for the metabolic furnace. *Although your body completely surrounds its digestive tract, food* <u>within</u> *the gullet and gut does not really get* <u>inside</u> *the body until it has crossed the wall of the intestines and been absorbed by blood capillaries or lymph ducts.* This passage

of materials across the intestinal barrier is highly selective
and finely regulated. Only small molecules—principally
water, amino acids, simple sugars, fatty acids, vitamins,
and minerals—penetrate the membrane under normal
conditions. Larger particles—including intestinal bacteria, or flora, and undigested proteins, carbohydrates, fats,
and roughage—are normally denied entry. If they acci-
dently breach the membrane, the body chemically recognizes them as "foreign" and attacks them with the full
force of its immune mechanisms.

That digestive microbes reside in the small intestine
is both usual and beneficial. Although they share all our
meals, these bacterial flora and fauna are necessary for the
complete breakdown of the food we eat. Fortunately, they
tend to consume only fractional amounts of our caloric
bounty and convert it in part to various vitamins (A, K,
E, and many of the B complex), which can be absorbed
and used. Although the amounts resulting from such synthesis "within but not inside" us are insufficient to fulfill
most human requirements for prolonged periods, they
provide an invaluable hedge against deficiency states, as
these "friendly beasties" continuously manufacture essential vitamins that are absorbed into our bloodstream irre-
gardless of diet. This vitamin failsafe mechanism probably
evolved as an important survival factor during periods of
famine. Today it protects against the manmade famine
of calorie-rich and vitamin-poor foods but clouds the issue
of your absolute personal need for dietary supplies of
vitamins.

Attempting to define fixed vitamin requirements and
actual vitamin intake is difficult. To know what concentrations of these nutrients remain in food after harvesting,
transportation, processing, and preparation is virtually
impossible. Most fruits and vegetables dropped into the
typical American market basket have been commercially
cleaned, peeled, and seeded; boiled, baked, dehydrated, or
fried; canned, bottled, boxed, or frozen. Similar "services"
have been rendered in the preparation of convenience
forms of meat, dairy products, and baked goods. Each

"time-saving" manipulation is destructive of vitamins. Exposure to air (oxygen), light, or heat physically and chemically disrupts such fragile molecules, causing them to lose essential biochemical properties. Harmful oxidation begins as protective peels, rinds, or skins are removed and vitamin-laden tissue, pulp, or flesh comes into direct contact with light and air. A sliced cucumber, pared potato, or carved steak becomes rapidly impoverished in this fashion. Heating is similarly destructive as it breaks many of the chemical bonds that maintain molecular integrity. Only the interior portions of cooked meats and vegetables are reasonably protected from such assault.

Food, subjected to multiple handling by anonymous hands, often enters the kitchen already depleted or compromised. Whatever vitamin content remains may be further eroded as the cook repeats and compounds the destructive practices already used by the processor. Excessive cooking and reheating, serving delays, prolonged freezer storage, slow thawing, and failure to seal prepared food from the ravages of light and air are particularly devastating culinary practices.

Although the vitamin content of your food is at best uncertain, there is a predictable disparity between the amounts you ingest and the concentrations you actually absorb. Losses occur because many vitamins remain locked in indigestible cells (provitamin A in raw carrots), unabsorbed for want of a proper fat solvent (vitamins A, D, E, or K), or unused because they exist in forms that cannot be metabolized by body cells (the vitamin B_3 of most breakfast cereals).

Under abnormal, but not infrequent, conditions both bacterial and dietary vitamin supplies may be diminished. Intestinal surgery, gall-bladder failure, parasitic infections, or the use of laxatives may limit your capacity to absorb these essential nutrients from the gut, while chronic diarrhea, antibiotics, and sulfanilamides may destroy necessary bacterial flora, interfere with normal digestion, and prevent both microbial and dietary supplies from reaching their target cells and tissues.

Vitamin Synergists and Allies

Once they have crossed the great intestinal divide and gotten into your body, many vitamins function as co-enzyme catalysts essential to all cells (B_1, B_2, B_6, B_{12}, folic acid, pantothenic acid, and biotin). Because they work synergistically, or as a team, the least effective or least concentrated of such catalysts determines a cell's efficiency. A similar interdependence comes into play as these same vitamins don different metabolic hats. Besides cooperative efforts in single cells, they function in the biochemical processes of specialized tissues and organs that yield substances, e.g. hormones, that coordinate and control the activities of the whole body. The human liver—a kind of biochemical clearinghouse—is the principal organ for such chemical integration. Its function relies upon an alliance or synergism among the various members of the B complex as well as vitamins A, C, D, and E, which also have multiple biochemical responsibilities. The kidney, brain, endocrine glands, bone marrow, intestines, pancreas, and muscle are similarly specialized organs whose unique biochemistry requires cooperation among vitamins to remain alive and to achieve their appropriate regulatory effects.

Chemical Antagonists, Adverse Conditions, and Increased Vitamin Demand

Although co-enzymes, as catalysts, are in theory unaffected by the chemical reactions they control and may be reused *ad infinitum,* vitamins are chemically fragile and susceptible to destruction by adverse conditions or chemical antagonists. A highly acidic or alkaline digestive tract or contact with powerful drugs, e.g. isoniazid, penicillamine, or broad-spectrum antibiotics, may destroy them—particularly members of the B complex—before they reach body cells and tissues. Other substances may interfere with the conversion of a vitamin to its co-enzyme or compete with it for a specific protein. Avidin, a component of uncooked egg whites, combines with B-complex biotin and renders it inactive, while thiaminase, a component of raw fish, splits vitamin B_1 into two inactive fragments. Sulfanilamides are so structurally similar to another member of the B complex that they challenge the vitamin by stealing its protein complement to create an inactive enzyme.

Although not destructive *per se,* the "empty calories" of the modern American diet place heavy demands on vitamin supplies and reserves. Since many calorie-laden foods do not contain equivalent co-enzyme complements, the latter must be drawn from tissue stores, which are limited—particularly for essential water-soluble co-enzymes. To achieve proper metabolism, any intake of protein requires a corresponding intake of A and B_3. A similar correlation exists between fats and vitamin E. Requirements for B_1 and B_2 escalate in response to the consumption of carbohydrates.

Protection of cells and tissues against the ravages of pollutants such as carbon monoxide, sulfur dioxide, and other waste chemicals; poisons such as petroleum distillates and solvents; and personal drugs such as caffeine, nicotine,[2] and alcohol[3] requires exceptional amounts of A, C, and E. These vitamins promote the health of the mucous membranes that act as a first line of defense against encroachment by such powerful environmental poisons. Their anti-oxidant, or oxygen-resistant, properties protect cells and tissues from breakdown caused not only by pollutant molecules but from destruction by ordinary— though toxic—metabolic by-products[4] as well. Effectiveness is buttressed by members of the B complex that main-

2. The stresses of tobacco usage deplete the body's supply and increase its demand for vitamin C. One-pack-a-day smokers commonly have only 50 percent of the tissue concentrations of C typical of non-smokers. Sub-clinical, or smokers', scurvy is the usual result.
3. Alcohol, as a pure carbohydrate, is entirely lacking in vitamins. The body metabolizes this calorie-rich but impoverished nutrient by cannibalizing its limited tissue stores or dietary sources of essential B-complex vitamins.
4. "Free radicals" are molecular fragments that "break off" from larger molecules during metabolism. They may cause severe tissue damage, as they are "free" to enter into disruptive chemical reactions often associated with cellular injury and aging.

tain optimum cellular metabolism and protect tissue against corrosive damage. Aspirin, oral contraceptives, and other drugs are potent physiological agents whose activities often increase metabolic demands and require a corresponding increase in vitamins to achieve their positive effects.

Vitamin Deficiency Disorders

Because vitamins are so intimately enmeshed in so many of your body processes and are so intricately linked with one another, biochemical injuries stemming from deprivation or depletion often express themselves in capricious ways and rarely result from lack of a single vitamin. Weakness, anxiety, malaise, and other vague complaints are typical of the universal cell impairment produced by deficiencies in the B complex. Symptoms may crystallize if one B-dependent organ or system is more vulnerable to insufficiency than another. Such variable susceptibility is a product of biochemical individuality, and similar deprivations may produce emotional aberrations in one person, diarrhea in a second, and a skin rash in a third. Similarly, lack of one or more of the vitamins may imperceptibly reduce the effectiveness of an organ and provide entrée to a disorder that has little obvious relationship to a deficiency. Reduced levels of A and C may affect liver function, restrict antibody formation, diminish tissue integrity, and limit white blood cell effectiveness, thereby exposing the body to a host of infectious diseases.

The absence of obvious correlation between symptoms of deprivation and lack of a specific vitamin can be illustrated as follows:

AFFECTED TISSUE	POTENTIALLY DEFICIENT VITAMIN(S)
Skin	A, K, B_2, B_3, B_6, biotin, C
Mouth	B_2, B_3, B_6, B_{12}, biotin, C
Intestines	B_1, B_3, B_6
Eye	A, D, K, B_1, B_2, B_3, C
Nervous System	B_1, B_3, B_6, B_{12}, folic acid
Blood (anemias)	E, B_2, B_{12}, biotin, folic acid
Heart and Blood Vessels	E, B_1, B_3, C
Skeletal System	A, D, C

Although the injuries caused by deficiencies can often be corrected with vitamin supplements, deprivation that has been extreme or prolonged may cause permanent tissue damage. Mild vitamin A insufficiency results in progressive but reversible night blindness *(nyctalopia)*. Extended deprivation may destroy nerve cells in the retina and produce an irrevocable decline in vision or even blindness *(xerophthalmia* and *keratomalacia).*

READER'S NOTE

The following catalogue is meant to provide you with a description of the various vitamins and their principal characteristics. Each profile is no more than a thumbnail sketch indicating how intimately and extensively vitamins are intertwined in the complex tapestry of human metabolism. You may simply wish to use this section as a reference and continue your reading with Chapter 5. Attempting to learn the biological properties of each vitamin—particularly those of the B complex—is apt to be confusing and is unnecessary.

THE FAT-SOLUBLE VITAMINS

Vitamins A, D, E, and K must be dissolved in fat before absorption through the intestinal membrane. Bile, produced by the gall bladder, and fatty acids from foods, the usual solvents, are important for getting these molecules into your bloodstream. Liver impairment or absence of dietary fats may lead to severe cell and tissue deficiencies of these vitamins. Because they can be stored in the body—particularly A and E—they may prove mildly disruptive following extended and exaggerated intake.

VITAMIN A

SYNONYM: Retinol

U.S. ADULT RDA: 5,000 IU/day

PRINCIPAL SOURCES: *Preformed:* Beef liver. *Provitamin form:* Apricots, broccoli, cantaloupe, parsley, turnips. (Carotene from plant foods is a vit. precursor. It is converted into vit. A by intestinal cells.)

ANTAGONISTS/ADVERSITIES/DEMANDS: Air pollutants; exposure to glare or strong light; nitrate fertilizers; mineral oil; dietary protein. *Preparation losses:* Heat of cooking and oxidation tend to destroy.

SYNERGISTS/ALLIES: Vit. D, E, C.

NORMAL FUNCTIONS: Vitamin A—

- maintains the integrity of mucous membranes lining the digestive tract, respiratory organs, salivary glands, and tear ducts. Health of these tissues is essential for resisting infections, allergies, and air pollutants.

- is required for the growth and repair of all cell membranes.

- participates in the formation of light-sensitive pigments needed for vision.

- maintains the health of the eyes, skin, and reproductive system.

- regulates the formation of cartilage and the synthesis of many hormones.

- must be present for protein metabolism in the liver.

- has essential co-enzyme functions in the retina, skin, liver, bone, and adrenal glands.

- may be stored in the liver, lungs, and kidneys for extended periods.

- aids in the detoxification of poisons.

DEFICIENCY DISORDERS: Lack of vit. A produces degeneration of eye tissue, specifically *nyctalopia* (night blindness) and *xerophthalmia* (lack of tearing), leading to *keratomalacia*. Blindness results from failure to form visual pigments and absence of eye lubricants. Growth retardation results from impaired hormonal, skeletal, and membranal biochemistry caused by a lack of vit. A.

OVERDOSE: Symptoms of excessive intake (lethargy, abdominal pain, headache, and profuse sweating) may follow prolonged ingestion of 100,000 IU/day or more for adults.

EXCEPTIONAL NEEDS:

- Diabetics and people with hyperthyroid metabolism have difficulty in converting provitamin carotenoids (plant sources) into usable A and may require supplementation, which can improve insulin production.

- Dietary increase in protein requires additional vit. A.

- By maintaining the integrity of mucous and cell membranes and because of its detoxifying action in the liver, vit. A helps protect the body during stress (injury, anxiety, surgery, poisoning, etc.) and promotes resistance to infection.

VITAMIN D

SYNONYMS: Calciferol, cholecalciferol, ergocalciferol

U.S. ADULT RDA: 400 IU/day

PRINCIPAL SOURCES: Vit. D forms on the skin as normal oils (cholesterols) are converted to the vitamin in response to the ultraviolet light of the sun; absorption follows. *Dietary:* Liver oils (e.g. cod and halibut), margarine, egg yolk, lard, yeast, shrimp, salmon, tuna, fortified milk.

ANTAGONISTS/ADVERSITIES/DEMANDS: *Drugs:* Cortisone, anticonvulsants, diphenhydantoin. *Preparation losses:* Oxygen and light tend to destroy.

SYNERGISTS/ALLIES: Vit. A, B_1, and B_3 increase tolerance of D, and vit. C helps prevent its oxidation. Calcium and D control bone formation.

NORMAL FUNCTIONS: Vitamin D—

- has essential co-enzyme functions in bone, kidney, liver, and intestinal metabolism.
- regulates the proper growth, hardening, and repair of bone by controlling the absorption of calcium and phosphorus from the small intestine.
- functions with parathyroid hormones to maintain proper mineral balance of calcium and phosphorus in body fluids and tissues (a hormonelike activity).
- maintains the hardness of teeth and bones.
- may be stored in the liver and skin.

DEFICIENCY DISORDERS: Lack of vit. D causes skeletal malformations and retarded growth in children *(rickets);* demineralizes and softens bones in adults, often producing a spontaneous break followed by a fall *(os-*

teoporosis and *osteomalacia);* softens teeth and makes them vulnerable to decay; reduces parathyroid activity; diminishes kidney function and muscle tone.

OVERDOSE: 3,000–4,000 IU/day in infants and 1,000 IU/pound/day in adults may lead to calcifying of kidneys, blood vessels, and skin.

EXCEPTIONAL NEEDS:

- Pregnancy draws heavily upon a woman's reserves in the formation of fetal bones.

- Absence of sunlight prevents formation of the vitamin.

- Softening bones and teeth are typical of the elderly, particularly women, and may often be related to vit. D deficiency.

- Toxic effects of lead and other heavy metals are partially offset by ingestion of D in conjunction with pharmacologic agents.

VITAMIN E

SYNONYMS: Tocopherol (alpha, beta, etc.)

U.S. ADULT RDA: 30 IU/day

PRINCIPAL SOURCES: Asparagus, broccoli, cabbage, chocolate, margarine, oils (corn, safflower, and soybean), peanuts, wheat germ, whole grains, yeast.

ANTAGONISTS/ADVERSITIES/DEMANDS: Oxidizing agents; food processing; rancid fats and oils; iron, when taken at the same time. *Drugs:* Oral contraceptives, thyroid hormone, mineral oil. *Preparation losses:* Heat, oxygen, and freezer storage tend to destroy.

SYNERGISTS/ALLIES: E, with vit. A, C, and B complex (particularly B_6, B_{12}, and folic acid), helps prevent, control, or cure certain forms of anemia. *Hormones:* Cortisone, testosterone, growth hormone (STH). *Minerals:* Selenium, manganese.

NORMAL FUNCTIONS: Vitamin E—

- is essential for the proper digestion and metabolism of polyunsaturated fats (vegetable oils), protecting them against oxidation and integrating them into cell and tissue membranes.

- ensures proper functioning of the circulatory, nervous, digestive, excretory, and respiratory systems as it maintains the integrity of cell membranes, e.g. of red blood cells and nerves, and membranous tissue of the intestines, kidneys, lungs, and liver.

- protects cells and tissues from damage caused by pollutants, toxic peroxides, and other free radicals formed by the ordinary metabolic breakdown of organic compounds. These molecules and fragments of molecules are implicated in cell degeneration and premature aging.

- promotes normal growth patterns and the body's ability to respond to stress.

- stimulates proper development and tone of the voluntary skeletal muscles and involuntary muscles of the heart and intestines.

- as a detoxifying agent and anti-oxidant may be involved in preventing or slowing the aging of body cells and tissues.

- may be stored in small quantities in muscle, fatty tissue, and the liver.

- requires bile or dietary fat for absorption (only 40 percent of dietary intake is typically absorbed from the small intestine).

- maintains the reproductive system in rats and other laboratory animals but has little or no effect on human sexual function.

DEFICIENCY DISORDERS: No clinical depletion diseases are known. Because of its role in protecting the red blood cell membrane, vit. E helps prevent various forms of anemia.

OVERDOSE: Because only minute quantities can be stored, there is little chance of toxicity. Extreme supplementation may increase blood pressure.

EXCEPTIONAL NEEDS:

- Increased dietary intake of polyunsaturated fats (vegetable oils and shortening) requires increased vit. E for their metabolism. Improved digestion of unsaturated fats resulting from supplementation may lower calorie requirements.

- Deficiency in E may account for the failure of low-cholesterol diets to significantly reduce the incidence of heart attacks and circulatory disorders.

- Because of its detoxifying effects, increased intake of E can help protect body cells from stress and premature aging.

- Pregnancy and lactation place considerable demands on a woman's limited stores of vit. E.

VITAMIN K

SYNONYM: Koagulations vitamin

U.S. ADULT RDA: None

PRINCIPAL SOURCES: Intestinal flora ordinarily produce the vitamin from foodstuffs in the gut. *Dietary:*

Green leafy vegetables (cabbage, kale, spinach), beef, pork, cauliflower, tomatoes, peas, carrots.

ANTAGONISTS/ADVERSITIES/DEMANDS: *Drugs:* Oral anticoagulants, e.g. dicumarol, Coumadin, and warfarin; antibiotics, e.g. penicillin and tetracycline; sulfonamides; mineral oil; aspirin and aspirin substitutes.

SYNERGISTS/ALLIES: Vit. A, C, and K in combination promote the health of red blood cells; vit. E.

NORMAL FUNCTIONS: Vitamin K—

- is a co-enzyme essential for the synthesis of protein clotting factors in the blood.

- is a liver co-enzyme required for energy metabolism and respiration.

- requires bile or dietary fat for absorption, whether supplied by intestinal bacteria or food.

- may be stored in small amounts by the liver.

DEFICIENCY DISORDERS: Hemorrhaging results from reduction in the vitamin K–dependent synthesis of various clotting factors in the liver. *Hypoprothrombinemia,* a tendency for bleeding, is the condition that results from deprivation.

OVERDOSE: Because of limited storage capacity, the possibility of toxicity is remote.

EXCEPTIONAL NEEDS AND PRECAUTIONS:

- Newborn infants may lack sufficient intestinal flora for essential vit. K production (particularly the premature) and often require supplementation.

- Because deficiencies often result from powerful and disruptive therapies or medical problems (poor intestinal absorption or surgery), supplementation requires a physician's supervision.

THE WATER-SOLUBLE VITAMINS

There are nine generally recognized B-complex vitamins (B_1, or thiamin; B_2, or riboflavin; B_3, or niacin; B_6, or pyridoxine; B_{12}, or cobalamin; folic acid; pantothenic acid; biotin; and choline). Three others (inositol, PABA, and B_{15}, or pangamic acid) have achieved limited acceptance. Letter and subscript designations, e.g. B_4, B_5, B_7, etc., were once applied to compounds no longer thought to have vitamin properties in man.

Members of the B complex and ascorbic acid (C) dissolve in water, are rapidly absorbed, circulate freely, are rapidly excreted, and must be regularly replenished since they are poorly stored in body tissue. Concentrations exceeding levels of cell or tissue saturation are quickly expelled in urine[5] or sweat, and ingestion of these vitamins in virtually any quantity is safe for healthy individuals. Because they collectively participate in so many biochemical processes, absence of one member of the group will often disrupt an entire metabolic process. However, deprivation or depletion of a single co-enzyme is highly unlikely as the water-soluble vitamins tend to occur together in foods,[6] and associated disorders often result from multiple deficiencies. As fragile molecules these vitamins are more readily destroyed by processing, storage, and food preparation than their fat-soluble counterparts.

---

5. The use of diuretic medications accelerates the loss of water-soluble vitamins.
6. Even if your goal is simply to fulfill U.S. RDA requirements, it is virtually impossible to get enough of the B-complex vitamins with your knife and fork unless you regularly eat liver, kidney, and other organ meats.

VITAMIN B₁

SYNONYMS: Thiamin, thiamine

U.S. ADULT RDA: 1.5 mg/day

PRINCIPAL SOURCES: Brewers yeast, beef kidney, ham, eggs, plums, prunes, raisins, wheat germ, whole-grain flour.

ANTAGONISTS/ADVERSITIES/DEMANDS: Physical and emotional stress; food additives (particularly nitrites and sulfites); baking soda; air pollutants; alcohol; dietary carbohydrates. *Drugs:* Antibiotics. *Preparation losses:* Heat, light, and water tend to destroy.

SYNERGISTS/ALLIES: Other B-complex vitamins (particularly B_2, B_3, B_6, B_{12}, and pantothenic acid); antioxidant vitamins C and E; growth hormone (STH).

NORMAL FUNCTIONS: Vitamin B_1—

- is an essential co-enzyme for all cells. It is necessary for the controlled release of energy from carbohydrate food molecules.

- is required for cellular synthesis of acetylcholine, the hormone that transmits impulses from one nerve cell to another.

- is a principal co-enzyme in liver chemistry.

- helps maintain the health of nerves, heart, muscle, and digestive tissue.

- promotes proper body growth and repair.

- as a water-soluble vitamin must be continuously supplied from dietary sources (minute amounts may be retained in heart, liver, kidney, and brain tissue).

DEFICIENCY DISORDERS: *Sub-clinical beri beri* may produce symptoms of fatigue, weight loss, appetite suppression, stomach upset, poor reflexes, weakness, memory loss, irritability, and/or depression before becoming *clinical beri beri,* which may occur in infants or adults as a severe neurologic disease—producing tissue swelling, or edema (wet form), and/or mental and motor dysfunctions (dry form), characteristic of acute alcoholism and schizophrenia.

EXCEPTIONAL NEEDS:

- Increased dietary ingestion of carbohydrates requires B_1 for proper metabolism. (Need depends on body weight, caloric intake, age, etc.)

- The chemistry of pregnancy and lactation increases demand for the vitamin.

- Many cardiac patients reveal only 50 percent of the tissue concentrations of B_1 characteristic of their non-cardiac counterparts.

- Alcohol, aging, allergies, surgery, and fever tend to elevate body requirements for the vitamin.

VITAMIN B₂

SYNONYM: Riboflavin

U.S. ADULT RDA: 1.7 mg/day

PRINCIPAL SOURCES: The liver, heart, and kidney of beef, pork, sheep, and veal; milk; brewers yeast; broccoli; eggs.

ANTAGONISTS/ADVERSITIES/DEMANDS: *Drugs:* Antibiotics, oral contraceptives. *Preparation losses:* Heat, light, and oxygen tend to destroy.

SYNERGISTS/ALLIES: Other B-complex vitamins; anti-oxidant vit. E; vit. A, B_2, and B_3 promote the health of eye tissues.

NORMAL FUNCTIONS: Vitamin B_2—

- acts as an essential respiratory co-enzyme in all cells, playing a critical role in the conversion of dietary protein to usable energy.

- in conjunction with vitamin A, maintains mucous membranes lining the respiratory, digestive, circulatory, and excretory tracts, while preserving the integrity of the nervous system, skin, and eyes.

- helps regulate the synthesis of essential growth (STH), metabolic (thyroxine), adrenal (ACTH), and pancreatic (insulin) hormones.

- helps control the growth and development of the fetus.

- must be converted to usable forms by the small intestine.

- may be stored in minute quantities in kidney, heart, and liver tissue.

DEFICIENCY DISORDERS: Severe personality disturbances result from interference with nerve-cell metabolism. Sub-clinical symptoms may include fatigue, loss of appetite, digestive upset, anxiety, and hypertension before deficiency produces clinical lesions of the lips, mouth, eyes, skin, and genitals.

OVERDOSE: Toxicity in humans has not been reported.

EXCEPTIONAL NEEDS:

- Reduced levels of B_2 in cells and tissues of the elderly may indicate that degenerative diseases are related to deficiency of the vitamin.

- The greater the dietary intake of protein, the greater the need for B_2.

- Liver damage resulting from B_2 deficiencies impairs normal function but may remain undetected for many years.

VITAMIN B_3

SYNONYMS: Niacin, niacinamide, nicotinic acid, nicotinamide

U.S. ADULT RDA: 20 mg/day

PRINCIPAL SOURCES: Intestinal flora may convert the amino acid tryptophan into B_3. Approximately 60 mg are needed to yield 1 mg of the vitamin. *Dietary:* Liver of beef, chicken, pork, sheep, and veal; roasted peanuts; swordfish; tuna; halibut; yeast.

ANTAGONISTS/ADVERSITIES/DEMANDS: Alcohol; physical and emotional stress; dietary carbohydrates. The B_3 of cereals, vegetable greens, seeds, and corn may be chemically bound into metabolically unusable forms. *Drugs:* Antibiotics. *Preparation losses:* Heat of cooking tends to destroy.

SYNERGISTS/ALLIES: Other B-complex vitamins (particularly B_1, B_2, B_6, B_{12}, pantothenic and folic acids); vit. A, C, D.

NORMAL FUNCTIONS: Vitamin B_3—

- forms a co-enzyme essential for the metabolism of carbohydrates, fats, and proteins in all cells.

- maintains normal rates of body growth and adequate energy supplies.

- promotes the synthesis of bile salts needed for the

digestion of fats and the absorption of fat-soluble nutrients (vit. A, D, E, and K).

- regulates the synthesis of hormones (thyroxine, insulin, and somatotropin, or STH).

- may reduce blood and tissue levels of the cholesterol and triglycerides associated with heart and circulatory diseases.

- functions particularly in the liver, skin, intestines, and spinal cord.

- may be stored in the liver, brain, and cardiac tissue in minute quantities.

DEFICIENCY DISORDERS: Clinical *pellagra* is a depletion disease whose symptoms include dermatitis (skin rash), dementia, and severe diarrhea. In contemporary America it is most frequently observed among alcoholics, diabetics, cancer victims, and sufferers from chronic diarrhea. Pre- or sub-clinical symptoms may include lassitude, mild skin rash, diarrhea, irritability, headache, false suntan, loss of memory, and appetite suppression.

OVERDOSE: B₃ is regarded as non-toxic in quantities less than 3–4 grams/day.

EXCEPTIONAL NEEDS:

- Large doses of B₃ may be used for the treatment of migraine headaches, *angina pectoris,* and other diseases requiring alteration in the diameter of blood vessels.

- Because of its role in promoting the metabolism of fats, the vitamin may help limit the buildup of cholesterol and triglycerides, which may in high concentrations cause heart attacks and circulatory disorders (cerebral hemorrhages, phlebitis, strokes, etc.).

VITAMIN B$_6$

SYNONYMS: **Pyridoxine, pyridoxal, pyridoxamine**

U.S. ADULT RDA: **2 mg/day**

PRINCIPAL SOURCES: **Liver of beef, chicken, and pork; brewers yeast; peanuts; herring; mackerel; salmon; soybeans; walnuts.**

ANTAGONISTS/ADVERSITIES/DEMANDS: *Drugs:* **Penicillamine, isoniazid, hydralazine, cortisone, oral contraceptives, levodopa.** *Preparation losses:* **Food processing, heat, and light tend to destroy (40–50 percent typically lost in kitchen handling).**

SYNERGISTS/ALLIES: **Other B-complex vitamins (particularly B$_1$, B$_2$, and B$_3$); vit. C; magnesium.** *Hormones:* **Epinephrine, norepinephrine.**

NORMAL FUNCTIONS: **Vitamin B$_6$—**

- acts as a co-enzyme in all cells and is necessary for their metabolism of protein and fats.

- acts as a co-enzyme for the synthesis of proteins from amino acids and regulates the synthesis of fats from dietary fatty acids.

- controls the formation or function of niacin, red blood cells, bile salts, and numerous hormones, including those involved with growth, human sexuality, and skeletal structure.

- helps prevent dental infection and cavities by maintaining the integrity of teeth and facial bones.

- functions as a co-enzyme in muscle, lymph, liver, and nerve tissue.

- is involved with maintenance of chemical balance among body fluids and regulates excretion of water, energy production, and resistance to stress.

- is retained by few tissues as 60 percent of the daily intake is typically excreted within 24 hours.

DEFICIENCY DISORDERS: Lack of B_6 produces symptoms associated with deficiencies in vit. B_2 and B_{12}, including sores of the skin, lips, and tongue. Anemia, convulsions, white blood cell dysfunctions, and hypertensive symptoms are characteristic of B_6 deficiency. Blood disorders and mental retardation are common effects of pre-natal deprivation.

OVERDOSE: Toxicity is rare and has only been observed at levels approaching 1 gram (1,000 mg)/pound of body weight/day.

EXCEPTIONAL NEEDS AND PRECAUTIONS:

- Tissue concentrations of the vitamin decrease with age.

- Increases in dietary protein and/or fat require a corresponding increase in B_6 intake for proper metabolism.

- Infants exhibiting symptoms of anemia, convulsions, and/or hyperactivity generally require B_6 supplementation for correction of their faulty blood and nerve chemistries.

- Oral contraceptives and cortisones tend to deplete supplies of B_6.

- Pregnant and lactating women generally require supplementation to compensate for fetal or infant demands.

- B_6 reverses the therapeutic effects of levodopa in the treatment of Parkinson's disease.

VITAMIN B_{12}

SYNONYMS: Cobalamin, cyanocobalamin

U.S. ADULT RDA: **6 mcg/day**

PRINCIPAL SOURCES: **Intestinal flora.** *Dietary:* **Liver and kidney of lamb, pork, beef, and veal; egg yolk; crab; salmon; sardines; herring; oysters.**

ANTAGONISTS/ADVERSITIES/DEMANDS: *Drugs:* **Aspirin and aspirin substitutes, codeine, chloramphenicol, oral contraceptives, neomycin.** *Preparation losses:* **Heat, light, and oxygen tend to destroy.**

SYNERGISTS/ALLIES: **Other B-complex vitamins (particularly B_1, folic acid, biotin, and pantothenic acid); vit. A, C, E.**

NORMAL FUNCTIONS: **Vitamin B_{12}—**

- **acts as a co-enzyme in all cells, assisting in the synthesis of nucleic acids (DNA and RNA), proteins, and fats from dietary raw materials.**

- **functions with folic acid to regulate the formation of red blood cells and genetic materials.**

- **additionally acts as a co-enzyme involved with essential liver, neural, kidney, heart, muscle, skin, and bone metabolism.**

- **maintains the health of nerve-cell membranes, tissue membranes, the intestinal tract, bone marrow, and growth hormones.**

- **may be synthesized by intestinal bacteria but requires "intrinsic factor" (produced by the stomach) for absorption to occur.**

- **is largely destroyed by processing and normal food preparation.**

- **is entirely excreted from the body within 6 days.**

DEFICIENCY DISORDERS: **Poor growth, pernicious anemia, disrupted carbohydrate metabolism, and degeneration of the nerves and spinal cord are typical effects** produced by B$_{12}$ deprivation. Known sub-clinical symptoms include memory loss, paranoia, and exaggerated fluctuations in mood. Psychosis may precede outright deficiency symptoms by many years.

OVERDOSE: There is no evidence for toxicity in man as injections of more than 1,000 mcg/day have produced no perceptible ill effects.

EXCEPTIONAL NEEDS:

- Vegetans (vegetarians who eat neither meat nor animal products) invariably experience B$_{12}$ deficiency without supplementation.

- Oral contraceptives elevate body requirements for the vitamin.

FOLIC ACID (B Complex)

SYNONYMS: Folacin, folate

U.S. ADULT RDA: .4 mg = 400 mcg/day

PRINCIPAL SOURCES: Intestinal bacteria synthesize small amounts of the vitamin. *Dietary:* Kidney, liver, and heart of beef, lamb, pork, and chicken; asparagus; bran; tuna; yeast.

ANTAGONISTS/ADVERSITIES/DEMANDS: Alcohol; physical and emotional stress. *Drugs:* Oral contraceptives, methotrexate, sulfonamides. *Preparation losses:* Heat, light, and oxygen tend to destroy.

SYNERGISTS/ALLIES: Other B-complex vitamins; vit. C. *Hormones:* Estradiol, testosterone, somatotropin (STH).

NORMAL FUNCTIONS: Folic acid—

- acts as an essential co-enzyme in all cells, participating in the synthesis of nucleic acids (DNA and RNA), choline, and enzymes necessary for all cell divisions.

- regulates the embryonic and fetal development of nerve cells.

- maintains the nervous system, intestinal tract, sex organs, white blood cells, and normal patterns of growth.

- is a constituent of genes and chromosomes in every cell.

- acts as a natural analgesic, or pain-killer.

- may be stored in minute quantities in the liver but is largely excreted from the body within 24 hours.

DEFICIENCY DISORDERS: Failure of proper nucleic acid synthesis results in numerous cell and tissue disruptions. Some forms of anemia (megoblastic, macrocytic, and pernicious) are common products of deficiency.

OVERDOSE: None reported.

EXCEPTIONAL NEEDS AND PRECAUTIONS:

- Folic acid may correct the red blood cell disruptions of pernicious anemia but may mask the neurological (brain) damage that must be corrected with vit. B_{12}.

- Anemia, reflecting deficiencies in iron, B_{12}, and folic acid, is common among pregnant women.

- Intestinal malfunction, cancer, pregnancy, and some blood disorders typically elevate the body's requirement.

- Vit. C may produce increased urination, which

can lower folic acid levels in the blood and other body fluids.

● The use of oral contraceptives typically increases the body's demands for the vitamin.

PANTOTHENIC ACID (B Complex)

SYNONYM: Anti-stress vitamin

U.S. ADULT RDA: 10 mg (Food and Nutrition Board estimate: 4–7 mg/day)

PRINCIPAL SOURCES: Brewers yeast; beef, pork, lamb, and chicken liver; eggs; herring; raw peanuts; bran.

ANTAGONISTS/ADVERSITIES/DEMANDS: Methyl bromide (insecticide fumigant used in storing and preserving foods). *Preparation losses:* Heat of cooking typically destroys at least 40 percent of the vitamin.

SYNERGISTS/ALLIES: Other B-complex vitamins; vit. A, C, E; calcium.

NORMAL FUNCTIONS: Pantothenic acid—

● acts as a co-enzyme essential for carbohydrate, protein, and fat metabolism in all cells.

● is required for the synthesis of hormones: acetylcholine in nerve cells, somatotropin (STH) for growth, and the adrenal hormones, which control numerous body functions.

● is required for the synthesis of essential body fats from basic fatty acids.

● plays an essential role in promoting the intake of amino acids, balancing tissue levels of water, and preventing infection.

● may be stored in minute amounts in liver, heart,

and kidney tissues (more than 30 percent is typically excreted within 24 hours).

DEFICIENCY DISORDERS: Although no specific disease is associated with depletion, deficiencies often increase susceptibility to infection and produce mental depression, physical weakness, reduced synthesis of bile salts, and disruption of normal nerve function. Loss of appetite, constipation, and fatigue are common sub-clinical symptoms preceding depletion.

OVERDOSE: Toxicity in man has not been documented and is improbable.

EXCEPTIONAL NEEDS:

- Pantothenic acid is routinely used to overcome post-operative shock and poisoning with curare or isoniazid, and may relieve symptoms of vertigo due to general debilitation.

- Because it strengthens white blood cells, the vitamin promotes wound healing and resistance to infection.

- Pantothenic acid may have anti-carcinogenic effects, is useful in treating cirrhosis of the liver, and promotes insulin production among marginal diabetics.

- Because of its normal metabolic functions, the vitamin helps counteract the injury produced by physical and emotional stress.

BIOTIN (B Complex)

SYNONYM: Vitamin H

U.S. ADULT RDA: .3 mg = 300 mcg/day

PRINCIPAL SOURCES: Intestinal bacteria synthesize fractional amounts of the vitamin. *Dietary:* Yeast, pork, liver, wheat, corn, mushrooms, salmon, chicken.

ANTAGONISTS/ADVERSITIES/DEMANDS: Raw egg white (avidin); choline. *Drugs:* antibiotics, sulfonamides. *Preparation losses:* Heat, light, and oxygen tend to destroy.

SYNERGISTS/ALLIES: Other B-complex vitamins (particularly B_2, B_6, B_{12}, folic acid, and pantothenic acid); vit. A, D. *Hormones:* Growth (STH), testosterone.

NORMAL FUNCTIONS: Biotin—

- regulates the metabolism of unsaturated fatty acids and participates in the synthesis of body protein, carbohydrate, and fat.

- maintains the sweat glands, nerve tissue, bone marrow, male sex glands, blood cells, skin tone, and hair quality.

- acts as a liver co-enzyme involved in at least four metabolic pathways.

- may be stored in liver tissue but is inactivated by rancid fats and choline.

DEFICIENCY DISORDERS: No specific depletion disease is known. However, biotin deprivation prolongs the effects of some protozoan infections.

OVERDOSE: Toxicity is not established.

EXCEPTIONAL NEEDS: None known.

CHOLINE (B Complex)

SYNONYMS: None common

U.S. ADULT RDA: None established. The Food and Nutrition Board considers choline a vitamin but lacks sufficient evidence to establish an RDA.

PRINCIPAL SOURCES: Some biochemical synthesis of the vitamin may occur within the body. *Dietary:* Beef liver, brewers yeast, eggs, lecithin, peanuts, wheat germ.

ANTAGONISTS/ADVERSITIES/DEMANDS: None specifically known other than those generally associated with related B vitamins.

SYNERGISTS/ALLIES: Other B-complex vitamins (particularly B_{12}, folic acid, and inositol); methionine (an amino acid).

NORMAL FUNCTIONS: Choline—

- is essential for the synthesis of fatty compounds that become components of all cell and tissue membranes.

- helps regulate the movement of substances across cell and tissue membranes.

- is required for the synthesis of acetylcholine, which transmits impulses from one nerve to another, and plays a critical role in memory functions.

- enables the liver to metabolize fatty deposits, which ordinarily concentrate in that organ and interfere with its biochemical efficiency.

DEFICIENCY DISORDERS: In at least ten species of animal, choline deficiency leads to fatty infiltrations of the liver and severe hemorrhages in kidney tissue. Similar disorders in man include cirrhosis, liver steatosis, and chronic hepatic disease. Evidence that choline supplementation relieves these human conditions is circumstantial.

OVERDOSE: The typical diet probably provides 500–900 mg of choline per day. No information is available concerning the amounts of the vitamin synthesized by the body. However, symptoms of toxicity have not been reported in man or animals.

EXCEPTIONAL NEEDS: None known.

VITAMIN C

SYNONYMS: Ascorbic acid, ascorbate, anti-scorbutic vitamin

U.S. ADULT RDA: 60 mg/day

PRINCIPAL SOURCES: Green peppers, parsley, guava, broccoli, Brussels sprouts, strawberries, citrus fruits.

ANTAGONISTS/ADVERSITIES/DEMANDS: Air pollutants and industrial toxins; smoking; alcohol. *Drugs:* Aspirin, anticoagulants, antidepressants, diuretics, indomethacin, prednisone, steroid hormones, warfarin. *Preparation losses:* Heat, light, oxygen, and leaching tend to destroy, while extreme water solubility often causes major depletion during cooking.

SYNERGISTS/ALLIES: Bioflavonoids and B-complex vitamins (particularly B_6, B_{12}, folic acid, and pantothenic acid); vit. K; C protects vit. A and E. *Hormones:* Testosterone, somatotropin (STH).

NORMAL FUNCTIONS: Vitamin C—

- regulates amino acid metabolism.
- helps maintain the strength and integrity of blood-vessel walls, particularly those of the capillaries.

- acts as an anti-oxidant that protects other vitamins and body tissues—particularly membranes—from the injury caused by poisons, pollution, and free radicals.

- promotes the body's absorption of the mineral iron.

- assists in the formation of bones, teeth, and cartilage.

- affects the health of all cell and tissue membranes. It promotes metabolism necessary for formation of essential body fats.

- maintains the adrenal glands and ovaries, ensuring their proper production of various hormones.

- plays a major biochemical role in regulating normal body growth, wound healing, and reactions to stress.

- stimulates the production of infection-fighting white blood cells.

- prevents conversion of food nitrites to cancer-causing nitrosamines.

- acts as an essential co-enzyme in the production of collagen, steroid hormones, pigment molecules, and the components of cell and tissue membranes.

- as a water-soluble vitamin, is readily excreted by the body and must be regularly replenished from the diet. (Small amounts may be stored in the adrenal glands.)

DEFICIENCY DISORDERS: Lack of proper intake or poor metabolism may weaken the intercellular cement that causes cells to remain close to one another. Adhesive failure makes cells and tissues vulnerable to infection and deterioration. Deficiency of vit. C weakens the fibers maintaining capillary integrity and causes easy, inexplicable bruising, hemorrhaging, and tissue swelling (edema). Such enervation undermines dental strength and invites bacterial infection (cavities and *gingivitis,* or gum deterioration). Lethargy and general malaise may result from reduced synthesis of adrenal hormones. Clinical vit. C depletion produces scurvy and eventual death.

OVERDOSE: Although as much as 6–10 grams of vit. C per day has been regularly ingested by many individuals, no evidence of toxicity has been demonstrated. Large amounts of the vitamin may promote urination, which has little or nothing to do with conditions leading to or aggravating gout and other kidney diseases. Digestive upset due to supplemental acidity may be counteracted with buffering substances or by using ascorbate forms of C. Prolonged high-level supplementation sometimes leads to diarrhea. (The binder or filler, rather than the vitamin, may be at fault.)

EXCEPTIONAL NEEDS AND PRECAUTIONS:

- Although vit. C does not seem to prevent the common cold, it evidently reduces the severity of symptoms, promotes general good health, and protects the body from injury caused by infections, trauma, stress, and aging.

- As a detoxifying agent the vitamin helps protect cells and tissues from poisoning by drugs (aspirin and barbiturates), pollution (carbon monoxide and cigarette smoke), alcohol, and radioactivity.

- By preventing the oxidation of essential fatty acids, the vitamin retards the formation of toxic free radicals associated with cellular aging.

- Because of its detoxifying and anti-oxidant effects, vit. C may interfere with laboratory tests—in particular, it may lead to a false positive reading for blood sugar.

- If a woman has supplemented her diet with C during pregnancy, her infant may require the vitamin to avoid scurvy-like symptoms of withdrawal after loss of contact with the maternal blood supply.

THE CONTESTED VITAMINS

Although traditional authorities do not classify them as vitamins, at least twenty compounds exhibit vitamin or vitaminlike properties in human metabolism. Recognition may be withheld for a number of reasons having little to do with a substance's activity as a co-enzyme. Some may be synthesized by intestinal bacteria. Others may occur so abundantly in so many foods that dietary deficiency is rare and escapes clinical detection. Yet others may yield identifiable symptoms that are difficult to relate to lack of the substance because too little of its biochemistry is fully understood. Whether such compounds are required in human nutrition is uncertain. That they are necessary for human metabolism is indisputable. Dietary need or absence of need probably depends on an individual's unique biochemistry. Among those vitaminlike substances whose classification is contested are a number of unquestioned metabolic utility and importance.

INOSITOL (B Complex)

This poorly understood B-complex vitamin concentrates in brain, liver, and nerve tissue. It is involved in reactions controlling the metabolism of fats and seems to play a significant role in reducing blood and tissue deposits of cholesterol while improving muscle tone and function. Although the mechanisms are unclear, these effects seem to depend on a synergism with biotin, choline, and vitamin E, while the presence of the vitamin seems essential for proper pantothenic acid function. A deficiency of inositol has been related to the nerve damage of muscular dystrophy, hardening of the arteries, and fatty degeneration of the liver, but the evidence for such effects is not conclusive. Beef brain and heart, brewers yeast, and wheat germ are rich food sources for the vitamin, but are not common components of the American diet. Most inositol is probably derived from intestinal bacteria, whose capacity to supply the compound may be impaired by antibiotics, mineral oil, diarrhea, and other digestive-tract disruptions.

PABA (B Complex)

Para aminobenzoic acid (PABA) acts as an essential co-enzyme in the metabolism of proteins and in the formation of red blood cells. It is a constituent of folic acid and stimulates production of that vitamin by intestinal bacteria. PABA is a pantothenic acid synergist. Because it is structurally similar to sulfanilamides, molecules of the vitamin and the antibiotic are metabolically competitive. That the side effects of sulfanilamides and deficiencies of PABA resemble one another is not surprising. Both can cause hypertension, anxiety, and digestive disorders. Although the vitamin occurs naturally in brewers yeast, wheat germ, and yogurt, PABA's partial synthesis by intestinal flora is used to deny its proper recognition.

PANGAMIC ACID[7] (B Complex)

Pangamate and vitamin B_{15} are synonyms for pangamic acid. It apparently functions as a co-enzyme involved in respiration, protein synthesis, and the regulation of steroid hormones. Because its principal effect is to increase blood and tissue supplies of oxygen, the vitamin may help detoxify pollutants, protect the liver, and extend life expectancy for individual cells, while promoting the activity of white blood cells and reducing susceptibility to infection.

Pangamic acid has not been identified as a vitamin since its need in human nutrition is not fully established. Its absence does not lead to any indisputable deficiency or disorder. Ignoring evidence of its co-enzyme functions,

---

7. N,N-Dimethylglycine.

the FDA threatens to brand the vitamin as an "additive" when included in food supplements. In France, Spain, Germany, Japan, and the USSR, the vitamin is regarded as essential and recommended allowances have been set at levels of 25–50 mg/day for adults. Symptoms of toxicity appear only at dosages 50,000–100,000 times greater than this amount. In this country supplementation with B_{15} is common among athletes and racehorses, in whom increased supplies of cell and tissue oxygen are desirable. According to recent but unconfirmed evidence, the vitamin may play a significant role in preventing, retarding, or curing heart disease, premature aging, senility, allergies, mild poisoning, neuritis, hypertension, hepatitis, and diabetes. Apparently B_{15} naturally occurs wherever B-complex vitamins are commonly found—principally in brewers yeast, organ meats, and whole grains.

BIOFLAVONOIDS

Vitamin P, flavones, and flavonols are general synonyms for the class of compounds known as the bioflavonoids. Rutin, hesperidin, tangeretin, nobiletin, and sinensetin are specific members of the nutrient group. Although the biochemistry is not fully understood, synergism between ascorbic acid and the various bioflavonoids helps maintain the blood capillaries, whose integrity is essential for the regulation of all substances entering or leaving the circulatory system. Failure of the minuscule capillaries typically results in edema, or tissue swelling, spontaneous hemorrhaging, and general disruptions of body function. Although bioflavonoids are concentrated in green peppers, tomatoes, apricots, rhubarb, and the pulp and rind of citrus fruits, periodic dietary deficiency may result from patterns of seasonal consumption and may cause or exacerbate the retention of tissue fluid associated with the menstrual cycle, occult bruises, hemorrhoids, or varicose veins.

A WORD ABOUT MINERALS

Minerals, like vitamins, may act as co-enzymes in numerous biochemical processes. Unlike their organic counterparts, these inorganic molecules are hardy in the face of physical and chemical abuse. They often prove toxic in excessive concentrations and must be used cautiously as food supplements. Although mineral deprivation or depletion will cause deficiency disorders—notably anemia due to a lack of iron—you are probably wise to be guided by U.S. RDA values for supplementation. Rely on dietary sources and water supplies for an added measure of metabolic insurance. (See Appendices A–D for further information about minerals.)

5

Your Vitamin Needs: An Alternative Viewpoint

Our studies at Harvard suggest that the average physician knows a little more about nutrition than the average secretary—unless the secretary has a weight problem. Then she probably knows more than the average physician.

— JEAN MAYER

Man is Nature's finest and most awesome creation. Since his emergence from relative ancestral obscurity more than 3 million years ago, he has gained ascendance over all other varieties of life. His unique intelligence, social capacity, and biochemical adaptability made him fit to compete with mammoth and mastodon. In succeeding ages these same qualities helped him tame and domesticate less formidable beasts, eliminating those that threatened his survival while he selectively bred and maintained those that assured his sustenance and security. In much the same way he bent vegetation to his will, cultivating varieties that fed him and his herds while destroying or discouraging those that lacked such usefulness. With his recent discovery of antibiotics and viral vaccines, he has subjugated the last of his biological adversaries. Having excelled other species in the rough-and-tumble struggle for survival, he now possesses absolute power to preserve or destroy any and all forms of life.

Although it took millions of years to achieve biological supremacy, man's pre-eminence was attained without benefit of vitamin supplements. You may wonder—more than four fifths of the way through the twentieth century —why anyone should think he now needs such assistance. In past eras and epochs, as the human race achieved comparative biochemical harmony with itself and its surroundings, the processes of species modification and adjustment were comparatively slow. Environmental forces such as weather, climate, and available food supply determined which organisms survived and multiplied or succumbed without issue. In modern times man has turned technological and social skills to immediate advantage but long-term detriment by dramatically altering the earth's ecological systems at so revolutionary a rate and in so radical a fashion that traditional patterns of species selection and adaptation have been severely impaired.

Profound interference with Nature's delicate balances began with the Industrial Revolution of the last century and escalated at a dizzying pace during the past thirty years. The result has been an increasingly befouled environment that places continuous, exaggerated, and abnormal demands on the genetic and metabolic apparatus of all living tissue. Although outward and visible signs of ecological contamination are easily identified, the internal havoc wrought by continuous interaction of body tissue with polluted air, water, and food is less easily perceived. Because toxification is insidious, cumulative, and pervasive, manmade ecological atrocities threaten the extinction of all species including that of the perpetrator himself.

Since there is scant chance that environmental purging and cleansing will be achieved in our lifetime, protection of vulnerable body tissue from environmental ravages must be a concern for everyone. Because vitamins help maintain the integrity of our biochemical defenses and neutralize the effects of metabolic poisons, their use—in quantities far exceeding those needed to prevent depletion disorders—is becoming a necessity in our ecologically deteriorating and chemically hostile environment.

A MATTER OF LIFE AND BREATH

Although the air we breathe today is as free as it ever was, we pay a high metabolic price for an inferior vapor that is very different from and less hospitable than that inhaled by our forefathers. It is now saturated with noxious chemicals, the long-accumulating waste products of heavy industry and the private automobile. Gaseous pollutants have encroached upon and poisoned the atmosphere in which man originated and evolved. Lead, nitrous dioxide, sulphurous gases, numerous hydrocarbons, carbon monoxide, and scores of other compounds now enter our lungs with every breath. Such toxic intruders subtly erode the delicate lining of eye, ear, nose, throat, and lung before absorption into the bloodstream. Their circulation to every cell, tissue, and organ of the body interferes with essential metabolic processes and impairs our health.

The liver is particularly susceptible to such pernicious and prolonged assault. Its normal function is to synthesize more than 1,100 different enzymes from various amino acids, vitamins, and minerals provided by our diet. Many of these resulting catalysts are involved in ridding the blood of toxins produced as by-products of ordinary cellular metabolism. The chronic intrusion of atmospheric pollutants places an abnormal burden on liver and other tissue as it increases the demand for enzymes essential to degrade these molecular interlopers. Although ample quantities of amino acids and minerals are usually available to meet additional needs, necessary vitamins—particularly the water-soluble varieties, which cannot be stored—are often in short supply. Absence or deficiency of any single co-enzyme is enough to retard the liver's cleansing function so that poisons continue to circulate to all body tissue, keeping it continually bathed in a sea of slight but persistent toxicity. Such mild internal poisoning inevitably produces a host of vague and undramatic ailments whose symptoms often include lassitude, exhaustion, and a general sense of ill health. After years of metabolic impairment by molecules foreign to every facet of our internal organs and external parts, injury to sensitive tissue may prove irreversible, and we become vulnerable to a host of infectious and degenerative diseases. Only by providing the liver and other body tissues with a generous and continuous reserve of *all* the vitamins can there be any assurance that they will be capable of nullifying the shock of contemporary chemical bludgeoning from a now alien environment.

PERSONAL POISONS

In our national pursuit of a higher standard of living we have unwittingly debased the quality of our lives. Not only do we foul our own nests by insisting on an inalienable right to pollution-causing automobiles, manufactured goods, and other privileges of conspicuous consumption but have in our passion for material wealth acquired personal lifestyles, consumer products, and *ersatz* foods that upset our body's internal equilibrium and damage its normal ecology.

A recent study by the National Institutes of Health indicates that more than 16 million American women—from Cannery Row to the White House—are dependent upon prescription barbiturates, tranquilizers, antidepressants, or sleeping pills. More than 2 million have a dual addiction to both mood-altering drugs and alcohol. Vulnerability to such personal and voluntary poisoning is an endemic problem not limited to the female of the species. It often involves an inability to cope with the physical and emotional pace, stresses, and pressures of contemporary life—problems that affect both men and women without regard to gender.

The purchase price of transient relief from tension provided by our modern opiates is exorbitant. It involves an initial and direct attack on cells of the liver, brain, and nervous system that produces the desired but unnatural anesthesia—a perverse mimic of genuine relaxation. Eliminating these molecular messengers of Morpheus requires heightened liver metabolism with its concomitant demand on all vitamin resources. Alcohol creates a secondary vitamin drain as its "empty" calories must be digested by catalysts whose co-enzymes are drawn from tissue stores or other food sources. If the habitual consumption of narcotics and intoxicants is compounded by the regular ingestion of caffeine or tobacco, the body is made to absorb cruel and unnatural biochemical punishment. Increased vitamin intake, proper nutrition, exercise, and rest can only partially offset such abuse.

GRAVE DIGGING WITH OUR TEETH

Abstaining from prescription medications, drinking, smoking, and caffeinated stimulants is no guarantee of the good life. We must eat to live, and it is a harsh reality of modern times that the typical American diet tends to subvert internal body chemistry and health. Because of our superior intelligence, sophisticated society, and technological prowess, we have increasingly ignored or forgotten the biological home truths of our evolutionary origin and development. Animal and vegetable cells derived from other living organisms are the natural foods to which we are biochemically attuned and adapted. Such "whole" nutrients in their raw state contain a majority, if not all, of the nourishment necessary for human life. When man began to cook his food, he acquired protection from infection but lost some nutritional elements to heat. Along with his invention of large-scale industry and its subsequent poisoning of the environment, he learned to process food in bulk—gaining efficiency and economic advantage at the expense of his physical well-being.

Today, instead of consuming nutritionally complete plant and animal tissues, we have been subtly converted to a diet of processed starch, sugar, vegetable oil, and animal fat. These contemporary "foods" are derived from energy storage sites in plant and animal bodies. They are rich in calories but lack the essential cellular nutrients of their parent organism. Without an adequate supply of these vital food elements—principally vitamins and minerals—metabolic efficiency and effectiveness are compromised. Because the modern supermarket dictates our bill of fare, we have little choice but to rely on substantial vitamin supplementation to compensate for the "benefits" of modern food technology and to guarantee that what we eat isn't undermining the fabric of our bodies and expediting our extinction.

Vitamin Parsimony: RDAs and U.S. RDAs

The doyens of the nutrition establishment who make periodic estimates of our vitamin requirements—the Food and Nutrition Board (RDAs) and the Food and Drug Administration (U.S. RDAs)—base their recommendations on amounts necessary to prevent outright clinical diseases such as scurvy, beri beri, and pellagra. Their adherence to such conservative and essentially negative values flies in the face of increasingly persuasive evidence that man's optimal intake of vitamins is many times greater than that required to stave off outright deficiency disorders.

Recent advances in biochemical research and technique have made possible precise and penetrating investigations of a cell's composition and activities. Current evidence provides a model that explains many of the profound changes that occur when vitamins are withheld from cellular nutrition. _Stage I:_ As external sources of supply are eliminated, ordinary metabolism continues until vitamin reserves are exhausted. _Stage II:_ Once total depletion is achieved, a cell makes radical, often heroic, adjustments to compensate for absence of such nutrient(s). Biochemical activity and efficiency are invariably reduced, and a cell may cannibalize its own nucleus, wall, and other structural elements to release vitamins for use in more critical metabolic processes. This twilight state of partial functioning can continue for long periods and may extend almost indefinitely if even small amounts of the deficient vitamin(s) are occasionally added to the diet. Although

Stage II damage may be irreversible, the addition of deficient vitamins in far larger quantities than normal can often restore full cellular health and activity. _Stage III:_ It is only after prolonged and total deprivation that complete biochemical catastrophe, breakdown, and cellular death occur.

While the foregoing applies to single microscopic units of which every individual is composed, there are good reasons to suppose that a similar pattern applies to the whole human body. If the generalization is valid, then most of us exist in a state of partial or Stage II vitamin deprivation for most of our lives. Because our diets normally provide us with marginal vitamin intake, few of us ever reach Stage III crises, but we continue to live in an uncomfortable limbo between outright sickness and genuine good health.

Such biochemical logic is attractive in an age when complaints of exhaustion, malaise, and non-specific ill health are common. That prolonged Stage II, or sub-clinical, vitamin deficiencies weaken body cells and cause their profound deterioration may well explain the dramatic increase in incidence of degenerative disease during the past twenty-five years. More than 80 percent of contemporary and killing disorders are the product of extraordinary tissue and organ deterioration or disrupted metabolism. Heart disease, circulatory disorders, cancer, diabetes, arthritis, and rheumatism may all follow as a consequence of prolonged, but correctable, vitamin deficiency.

To suppose that modern man survives on subsistence levels of vitamin intake gains support from the kind of time-honored evolutionary evidence that has long established his historical relationship to other organisms. Nineteenth-century comparisons of anatomical similarities and differences between various species provided Darwin with his basis for the Theory of Evolution. His fundamental ideas were confirmed in the twentieth century through chemical analysis and comparison of the cells and tissues of different organisms. The greater the similarity in body chemistry, the closer is the evolutionary affinity between species and the more recent their descent from a common ancestor. Our nearest biological relatives are the primates and great apes. Unlike most other more distantly related animals, neither man nor monkey can synthesize his own vitamin C. That the normal dietary intake of ascorbic acid by our closest ancestral kin exceeds our officially recommended dietary allowance by more than a factor of one hundred suggests that proponents of large-dose vitamin C nutrition are more than mere charlatans and quacks. Comparison of our officially recommended allowances for the other vitamins and the amounts required by primate metabolism suggests a similar, though less dramatic, disparity between prescribed intake and actual need for optimum biological function.

Although society has not rigorously tested the effects of massive vitamin ingestion on humans, Nature has repeatedly done so with her less sophisticated offspring. Animals in the wild naturally select foods rich in vitamins and tend to reject inferior alternatives unless faced with starvation. This innate sense of dietary body wisdom has been lost by man after centuries of industrialized civilization and by his herd animals after thousands of years of domestication. It has only been in recent decades that breeders, trainers, and farmers have recognized the value of providing their animals with vitamins in amounts far exceeding those necessary to assure "adequate" health and freedom from deficiency diseases. Optimal growth, resilience, and fitness seem to occur at levels corresponding to those proposed by responsible advocates of human supplementation. That man with all his scientific sophistication has recognized the importance of vitamins for his livestock but not for himself is one of the most tantalizing puzzles of the age.

Although we humans got into the twentieth century without the assistance of vitamin supplements, we did so before our food had been drained of essential nutrients and prior to any threat of ecological Armageddon. At this time of sharply reduced dietary supply and dramatically increased bodily demand, it makes sense to maximize the chances for good health by adding vitamins to our diets with reason, moderation, and a clear understanding of what supplementation can be expected to accomplish.

VITAMINS AND THE AMERICAN MEDICAL OLIGARCHY

That government health agencies and the orthodox medical establishment continue to scoff at the significance of optimal vitamin nutrition is a natural cause for concern to anyone considering vitamin supplementation. There is wisdom in caution. However, it is important to remember that the history of science and medicine is littered with the corpses of academic experts who rejected new and valid ideas that contradicted their notions of scientific truth.

After years of jeering at those who have added vitamin C to their diets, the FDA is about to order addition of the vitamin to all meats treated with nitrites. Evidently, ascorbic acid is one compound that can safely prevent conversion of these preservative molecules to cancer-causing nitrosamines. While this albeit tardy recognition of vitamin C is encouraging, it can provide little comfort to those who have religiously adhered to the governmental party line and have exposed themselves to carcinogenic foods. Because the FDA contemplates no comparable vitamin prophylaxis against the nitrogen-containing fertilizers used in growing our fruits and vegetables, it is clear that the individual must continue to protect himself against biochemical subversion from his officially sanctioned diet.

Although increasing numbers of medical practitioners are rebelling against the anti-vitamin orthodoxy of the American Medical Association and other hidebound professional organizations, the average physician of today is apt to know no more about nutrition—let alone vitamins—than his secretary. The reasons for such professional ignorance are the unfortunate result of our ordinarily democratic society's having allowed its health-care system to fall into the hands of a centralized, one-party dictatorship. The absolute and autocratic power of the FDA and the AMA has converted American medicine into a kind of state religion that promotes orthodox thinking and stifles all dissent. Disaffected by the failure of vitamins as "wonder drugs," the health-care establishment has turned its back on the importance of these compounds as nutrients rather than as medications. It has been left to the more receptive and flexible layman, independent research scientist, and non-conformist physician to recognize the important distinction between food and drug.

The All-or-Nothing Approach to Health

Although the existence of illness was once viewed as medicine's failure to fulfill its obligation to prevent disease, this attitude has undergone a subtle but radical change in modern times. The contemporary physician can only be expected to care for or cure a sickness, not to keep it from happening. The burden for maintaining personal health now falls squarely on the shoulders of each individual, while responsibility for relieving or ameliorating disease rests with his medical doctor. This division of labor is proper and logical since we—not our physicians—daily determine the personal habits that will either support or subvert our physical well-being.

Because he is primarily trained and equipped to intervene in crises that occur when the body breaks down in the face of physical injury, microbial invasion, or physiological malfunction, the conventional M.D. tends to view his patients as either "sick" or "well." This "all-or-nothing" approach to the individual leaves little time or inclination for anything but emergency care. The brusqueness, haste, and inaccessibility of the typical physician in non-crisis situations is frustrating to the average patient, who expects a far more scrupulous monitoring and supervision of his physical health than the brief scrutiny he normally receives. Disparity between the limits of a doctor's capabilities and his client's expectations often leads to antagonism that is resolved by the practitioner's prescribing a powerful, often irrelevant, drug or even surgical procedure to satisfy his patient's demands for attention. This misapprehension can have damaging, if not tragic, results. More than 50 percent of physicians consulted about the common cold dismiss their patients with antibiotics—drugs that have no effect on the viral cause of the disease but which may produce severe allergic reactions, even death. In a similar fashion, addictive barbiturates are routinely prescribed for vague complaints of tension and sleeplessness, while disruptive diuretics or amphetamines are commonly ordered to counteract listlessness or "assist" in weight reduction. Iatrogenic, or physician-caused, disease accounts for more than 160,000 deaths per year from prescription medications and for more than 2.5 million unnecessary operations that annually lead to 12,000 fatalities.

To expect our physicians to prevent any but infectious diseases or to enrich our physical well-being—except in times of acute bodily crisis—is unreasonable. As a group, medical practitioners enjoy no greater life expectancy nor better health than the average man. They are prone to all of the degenerative disorders, chronic sickness, and detrimental lifestyles of the age. When it comes to the theory and practice of good health, the layman and the professional are on equal ground. Failure of the physician to achieve exemption from illness is not surprising in light of the bias of his training.

Medical Schools:
Nutritional Ignorance in the Groves of Academe

In recent decades medical school curricula have been so standardized that education in one institution virtually duplicates that in every other. Although there are undeniable advantages to ensuring uniform excellence among the nation's physicians, such homogenization tends to produce cookie-cutter training, theory, and practice that allow no exception to rigid and revered principles. Because the technology is now so vast and the range of information so great, modern medical students must turn themselves into automatons whose every waking hour must be spent in achieving prodigious feats of memory at the expense of reflective thinking and questioning. That young malleable minds can master the pharmacology of today's analgesics, anesthetics, diagnostics, soporifics, tranquilizers, vaccines, and other medications is a tribute to the retentive powers of the human brain. Such incredible emphasis on the chemistry of drugs can only condition the medical neophyte to rely heavily on nonbiological therapies throughout the course of his subsequent career and practice. Because of his training, it is easy to forget that most of the drugs he prescribes will do no more than temporarily mask the symptoms of a patient's illness. They rarely strike at the core of a disease, let alone prevent it. People do not suffer from tension because they failed to take their tranquilizer, clog their arteries with cholesterol because of a lack of an anticoagulant medication, or develop arthritis because of an unfulfilled need for aspirin. Yet this year's medical graduate will predictably use such drug regimens to relieve symptoms rather than cure diseases for the next forty years.

Because medical training must be so condensed and compacted, the current course of study allots no more than cursory attention to the role of nutrition in health and disease. A student's brief encounter with the biochemistry of food and metabolism is excessively theoretical and provides no practical understanding of how the food we eat profoundly affects every body part and process throughout our lives. Although the characteristic symptoms and classical cures for vitamin depletion disorders are learned, they are acquired more as relics of medical history than as meaningful tools for modern therapy. Subclinical vitamin deficiencies receive little, if any, consideration. As a result, new physicians—like their predecessors —will neglect to examine patients for vitamin deprivation. They don't know how to do so and will find it easy to overlook or deride this common, if unfamiliar, biological phenomenon.

Vitamins Are <u>Not</u> Drugs

Most drugs are powerful chemical agents as alien to human tissue and metabolism as the noxious and toxic pollutants of our contemporary environment. They often achieve their effects by poisoning or otherwise disrupting normal body processes to achieve a desired but temporary relief from symptomatic distress. In carefully controlled quantities anesthetics, pain killers, tranquilizers, barbiturates, and other soporifics interfere with the brain and nervous system by toxifying and subsequently inhibiting usual functioning. If concentrations of these foreign molecules are even moderately excessive, they will more than deaden pain, induce sleep, or produce relaxation. They will kill, and their use must be meticulously restrained and professionally monitored with the benefits of central nervous system depression constantly weighed against the risk of death or permanent injury. Antibiotics interfere with the metabolism of foreign bacteria. Their catalysts of destruction are as foreign to the body as the invading microbe and may stimulate the body's defenses to attack and destroy its own antibiotic-saturated tissues. Such allergic, or anaphylactic, reactions unintentionally kill more than thirty thousand Americans every year. Another class of drugs, the analgesics, help to reduce painful swelling and inflammation—particularly that of arthritis and rheumatism—by suppressing the body's immune response. Repeated use of even common non-prescription pain-relievers such as aspirin can cause severe internal hemorrhages, destroy kidney tissues, and interfere with digestion. Only hormones may be considered natural medications whose presence in the body is normal. The vast majority of other drugs may be thought of as molecular lone wolves—predatory interlopers that pass rapidly through various regions of the body, hopefully achieving some good without permanently damaging the delicate ecology of the tissue they have invaded.

That "knowledgeable" health-care officials and "responsible" physicians have attempted to equate vitamins

—in any quantity—with drugs betrays a fundamental ignorance of both pharmacology and nutrition. Vitamins are not drugs. They bear no chemical or functional resemblance to such compounds. *Vitamins are foods*—nutrient molecules like the protein from a steak, starch from a potato, or sugar from an apple. Required by every human cell, their presence—unlike that of drugs—is essential for life and the absence of any one leads to death. As integral components of metabolism, they are chemically native, not alien, to the body and function cooperatively with one another to fulfill the biochemical business of life. Shortage of even a single member of the vitamin family reduces the effectiveness of the others and impairs the overall metabolic efficiency of any deprived cell, tissue, or organ. In contrast with nonbiological compounds, failure to maintain adequate concentrations of vitamins or any other nutrient results in varying degrees of starvation.

While even slight elevation in the concentration of a drug may turn its potential for good to evil, increased ingestion of vitamins even to levels of tissue saturation is arguably beneficial. Once maximum concentrations have been reached, any excess of the water-soluble varieties is excreted, while surpluses of fat-soluble forms are stored for future use. The much-touted dangers of immoderate vitamin intake—particularly for A and D—are ludicrous when compared with the effects produced by overdosages with drugs. The former occur only when either of the two vitamins is consumed in wildly exaggerated quantities for long periods of time. They produce only mild symptoms of distress, which disappear rapidly when supplementation ceases. The latter maim—often permanently—or kill.

Vitamin Nutrition and Disease

To assume that health is a kind of blind lottery in which all the participants have equal chances for success or failure is irrational. Biochemical resilience determines our susceptibility to disease. It is the forever-evolving product of continuous interaction between hereditary and environmental factors in our lives. Although we can do little to alter our genetic makeup, polluted environment, or past medical history, we can and do make daily choices that enhance or deny our potential for physical well-being. A well rested, exercised, and relaxed body that is free from dependence on artificial stimulants and depressants is obviously more resistant to infection and decay than one that is overwhelmed by stress, tension, and fatigue complicated by addiction to alcohol, caffeine, or tobacco. Whatever personal choices we make in honoring or abusing our body's innate capacities, none is biologically more important in determining its current health and future stamina than the quality of our daily diet. We are and we become what we eat.

Although few Americans are in danger of getting too few calories with their knives and forks, freedom from hunger is no guarantee of nutritional well-being. There are many grades of dietary excellence, and each profoundly affects the health of the body it supports. As a nation, we tend to be overfed and undernourished since most of us make food choices that promote both caloric *mal*nutrition and varying degrees of vitamin starvation. Because we fill our plates with refined carbohydrates and fats at the expense of their nutritionally whole alternatives and body-building proteins, our dietary supply of metabolic fuels consistently exceeds physical demand, and the surplus is regularly stored as fat. Caloric gluttony combined with protein deprivation in many makes us an overweight people whose excess poundage places life-threatening strain on the health of heart, kidneys, liver, and other body tissue. Because the symptoms of such caloric malfeasance are both physically obvious and socially undesirable, more than half of the adult population makes at least one yearly attempt to shed its excess personal baggage. Unless protein consumption is maintained, while caloric reduction is achieved by cutting fat and carbohydrate intake, weight loss will be indiscriminate—reducing not only deposits of fat but also the size of critical protein-containing muscle and organs as well. Such aggravated nutritional assault on the fabric of the body can only undermine its integrity and

exacerbate conditions of a more subtle and devious malnutrition that is typical of most Americans.

Whether we are overweight, underweight, or of "normal" avoirdupois, we are all composed of trillions of cells,
each requiring a continuous supply of nutrients. Proteins,
carbohydrates, and fats are the essential molecular building blocks and sources of energy necessary to fabricate,
power, and maintain each cell. They are useless without
the assistance of vitamin and mineral co-enzymes that
disassemble and rearrange raw nutrients before integrating their component amino acids, simple sugars, and fatty
acids into the cell's biochemical architecture and activity.
Even under the best of biological conditions, the cells of
our body must compete with one another for a full measure of molecular raw materials and essential catalysts.
Since more than 40 percent of the food now consumed in
this country has undergone processing and been stripped
of most—if not all—of its original vitamin complement,
the struggle for nutritional survival among the cells and
tissues is intense. Most capture enough of their vital co-
enzymes to remain alive but in marginal health. This state
of borderline vitamin starvation predisposes all cells to
premature deterioration and invites infection by viral and
bacterial agents. Because relative tissue fitness is a feature
of our unique biochemical individuality, the cells and tissues most vulnerable to cellular malnutrition may vary
enormously and produce very different symptoms from
individual to individual. Similar sub-clinical deficiencies
may lead to failing eyesight in one, decaying teeth in another, and arthritis in yet a third. Although millions of us
are "at risk" and vulnerable to the ill effects of prolonged
deprivation, vitamin malnutrition can be corrected and
many of its injuries reversed.

Although a nutritional approach to the prevention
and treatment of disease has long been resisted by the
medical establishment, the increasing incidence of degenerative illnesses clearly related to prolonged nutritional
folly has forced professional reappraisal of this intransi-

gent position. That an optimally nourished body is the one most resistant to infection, decay, and malfunction makes good biological sense. Unless an individual's own chemistry can respond to the threat of disease, all of a physician's wonder drugs and surgical skills are of little use. The heroic techniques that maintain life in a clinical vegetable are awesome, but offer little comfort or hope for a body that is no longer capable of sustaining itself. Cautious recognition of this fact has led the medical profession to proclaim a war on dietary cholesterol as the principal villain of heart and circulatory disease.

During the past ten years a nutritionally responsive and concerned public has dutifully reduced its consumption of cholesterol-laden animal fats, replacing them with more liquid vegetable shortenings and oils. The anticipated elimination of cardiac disorders has failed to materialize. Professional ignorance of vitamin metabolism may be at fault. Although solid deposits of cholesterol undoubtedly reduce the diameter of blood vessels, impair circulation, and help cause heart attacks, elimination of the molecule from the diet does not eliminate it from the body. In the absence of dietary supplies, the liver will convert varying quantities of polyunsaturated vegetable oils to cholesterol, which is needed for normal biological functioning. Only in the presence of ascorbic acid (vitamin C) and tocopherol (vitamin E) will the body metabolize plant fats to appropriate amounts of cholesterol and convert the remainder to less deleterious substances.

A similar nutritional confusion surrounds the cardiac's intake of refined starches, which tends to be much greater than that of the typical non-cardiac. Failure to produce remission of disease with a low-starch diet has proved frustrating to physicians. They often discount or overlook the prolonged effects of excessive carbohydrate intake, which placed an inordinate drain on the patient's dietary supplies of the B-complex vitamins (particularly thiamin, or B_1) required to metabolize refined starches and sugars. Although the dietary stress may be removed by minimizing carbohydrate ingestion, an acquired dependence on large amounts of the vitamin probably remains, and ignorance of the need may well maintain disease conditions.

Uncertainty about or ignorance of vitamin nutrition is typical of the medical profession today. Your dentist or periodontist may urge you to supplement your diet with vitamin C to restore weakened and bleeding gums before the appearance of tooth decay and jaw deterioration. Your internist may object that such therapy will upset the chemistry of your kidneys and produce acidic conditions that lead to gout, while your urologist may tell you that gout is caused by uric, not ascorbic, acid and hold no strong opinion about the value of vitamin supplements. Since our physicians have been slow to recognize the importance of nutrition and slow to resolve the current contradictions in their thinking about its role in preventing disease, we as individuals must continue to exercise our nutritional freedom of choice and good common sense in maintaining and promoting our bodily health.

Because we live in an age of increased demand and reduced dietary supply, it is undoubtedly wise to maximize our chances for good health by adding vitamins to our diets in safe quantities that not only prevent depletion disorders but also ensure optimal metabolic function. The time to begin such enrichment is long before the usual appearance of chronic and degenerative diseases. By beginning supplementation early we may achieve maximum physical rewards with a minimum of personal risk.

MINIMAL, RECOMMENDED, OR OPTIMAL DAILY HEALTH

Our personal vitamin requirements are unique. They cannot be predicted by committee or established by health agency decree. They distinguish us from all other individuals and are as idiosyncratic as the shape of an earlobe or the pattern of a footprint. Because our biochemical demands are so distinctive, it is a pity that this age of sophisticated medical hardware has not produced a vitamin equivalent of the stethoscope, blood-pressure cuff, or oral thermometer. If we could measure the metabolic efficiency of vitamin metabolism as a machine now monitors the activities of the heart, or determine vitamin levels in the body as laboratory analysis now reveals the concentration of sugars in the blood, we could know our exact vitamin status and needs with far greater certainty than is currently possible.[1]

Despite the absence of hard and fast personal data, there can be little doubt that our body's demand for vitamins can be fulfilled at varying levels of nutritional quality. At least three requirement values for each vitamin have particular relevance for each of us. These significant quantities are not the same for any two people or fixed and permanent for any one. They change for each of us in response to biochemical modifications that result from constant interaction between the hereditary and environmental factors in our personal lives. Past medical history, genetic heritage, degree of physical activity, rate of metabolism, stage of body maturity, and the composition of our diets are prominent variables that help determine the peculiar scale of our nutritional needs. At the lower limit is that <u>minimal concentration</u> of a vitamin necessary to keep the body alive. At the upper limit is an <u>optimal quantity</u> that ensures maximum biochemical efficiency and effectiveness. Between the two extremes is a value that should guarantee freedom from a vitamin-deficiency or depletion disease without having any necessary relationship to the quality of our unique metabolic processes.

In establishing its original proposals for the enrichment of staple foods in the early 1940s, the Federal Government promulgated its educated guesses about the minimum daily requirements (MDRs) thought necessary to keep a majority of the quick from the dead. More than twenty years later these subsistence figures were replaced

---

1. See Appendix A for information about newly developed tests your physician or dentist can order to determine your personal vitamin and mineral status.

by slightly more generous estimates, which are suggested or recommended daily vitamin allowances (U.S. RDAs) that *should* protect the average, though mythical, American from such diseases as rickets, beri beri, scurvy, or pellagra.

The contemporary decline in quality of our physical environment and food supply coupled with advances in biochemical understanding have led many research scientists, practicing physicians, and nutritionists to advocate dietary enrichment at levels intended to achieve optimal metabolic activity. The principal intent of such supplementation is to saturate body cells and tissues with *all* of the essential vitamins so that the relative lack of a single vitamin becomes a biochemical impossibility. It is only when we supply cells and tissues with overload quantities of their required co-enzymes that the body can compensate for reversible damage caused by prior vitamin starvation and begin to function at peak efficiency and capacity. *It seems impossible to elevate co-enzyme levels beyond an individually fixed and optimum concentration: Innate biochemical wisdom apparently prevents cells and tissues from absorbing more of the various vitamins than they can effectively use.* This built-in mechanism provides us with an ideal biological regulator of our optimal requirements as it automatically adjusts and adapts the body's vitamin metabolism to maintain maximum efficiency at all times and under all conditions. Our responsibility is to keep it functioning by providing ourselves with liberal supplies of all the vitamins so that tissue saturation and optimal function may be assured.

Megavitamin Myth and Reality

In recent years a veritable verbal whirlwind has swirled about the theory and practice of so-called "megadose" vitamin therapy. The adjective "megadose" is a singularly misleading term when applied to vitamin supplementation. The prefix "mega" multiplies the number of the noun it modifies by one million, and a "dose" is any specified amount of a medicinal agent or drug. Vitamins are foods, not drugs, and what could be more absurd than to speak of a dose of protein, carbohydrate, or fat? Or vitamin? Because the public is aware that even moderate increase in the prescribed intake of a prescription or a non-prescription drug may be harmful or lethal, we are officially encouraged to associate people who consume any more than the all-American U.S. RDA for a particular vitamin with "druggies," dope fiends, and addicts. No one —not even the most ardent vitamin advocate or enthusiastic research chemist—suggests supplementation at levels remotely approaching a million times the amount of any RDA. That their recommendations for attaining tissue saturation with a few of the vitamins exceed FDA standards by multiples in the hundreds is evidence for officialdom's indifference to optimum nutrition rather than the advocate's irresponsibility.

Legitimate confusion does surround the various possible levels of vitamin enrichment in less than "megadose" quantities. Concentrations necessary to attain tissue saturation for most people are considerably lower than those used by some research physicians, whose experiments with massive supplementation have reputedly cured or ameliorated such severe mental or physical disorders as schizophrenia, chronic heart disease, acute alcoholism, and migraine headache. The therapeutic use of vitamins in this medical context is based on the reasonable biochemical assumption that some individuals have either a genetic or an acquired need for vitamins in excess of that necessary for tissue saturation among a vast majority of the population. A number of inherited nutritional disorders that require either the dietary elimination or exaggerated intake of a specific nutrient are well documented, and the possibility that man's more recalcitrant diseases may be caused by an acute vitamin deficit is not illogical. Although reports of spectacular success with massive vitamin regimens receive sensational media coverage, most of these cures have not been scientifically substantiated, duplicated, or proved beyond reasonable doubt.

Vitamin Miracles and Mirages

The catalogue of benefits ascribed to vitamins is dazzling. Promises that supplementation can cure or prevent every human malady from graying of hair to grinding of teeth are grist to the mill of quasi-medical journals, popular magazines, the daily press, and an impressionable public. Compensation for individual and undetected sub-clinical vitamin deficiencies *can* help lower cholesterol levels, improve vision, increase energy, relieve hypertension, counteract environmental poisons, bolster resistance to both degenerative and infectious diseases, retard aging, and lengthen life. Such impressive effects result from meeting a body's unique and previously unfulfilled requirements for vitamins at optimal nutritional levels. To expect—as enthusiasts often suggest—that supplementation will confer uniform or even predictable advantages on every individual is foolhardy. Personal health is the product of a complex equation that delicately balances many factors of which vitamin nutrition is but one of the critical variables. The only certain value of supplying your body with generous amounts of all the vitamins is that a relative deficiency of these essential nutrients will *not* be an impediment or limiting factor to achieving and maintaining good health.

For some of us vitamin supplementation at any level is unnecessary although potentially desirable. The individual who practices wretched dietary habits but remains in prime fettle, perennially free from disease, is a remarkable but not unfamiliar figure. He belongs to a segment of the population whose inherited biochemical requirements are minimal and easily satisfied by prevailing foodstuffs and environmental conditions. The addition of vitamins to his diet can help ensure continued good health and provide him with a margin of metabolic protection as he ages. For the vast majority of us, who are not so fortunately endowed, vitamin supplementation at optimal levels provides no sure immunity from disease, deterioration, or aging and guarantees no fixed, absolute, or certain rewards. It *does* maximize at least one critical nutritional factor that promotes our health and well-being while posing a minimum of risk if practiced with intelligence and caution.

Optimum Personal Allowances (OPAs)

Because its biochemical uniqueness determines the body's metabolic requirements for various nutrients, there are as many different optimal levels of vitamin intake (OPAs) as there are people. In the absence of precise and accurate techniques for measuring the quantities of vitamins in foods; degree of absorption into the bloodstream; concentrations in body tissues, cells, and fluids; or actual vitamin needs, the OPA values used here (pages 154–155) are no more than guidelines for helping achieve optimal vitamin nutrition in a short period of time. By exceeding —but not unduly exaggerating—the body's probable capacity for absorbing and utilizing the various vitamins, your metabolic machinery can operate maximally, employing exactly those vitamin quantities it needs while rapidly excreting any excessive amounts of the water-soluble forms and storing any surplus of the fat-soluble varieties. For supplementation to achieve its desired effects, it is essential that your vitamin intake be—

- *Comprehensive:* Because vitamins work cooperatively, their rational use requires that all be taken together in balanced concentrations. No vitamin-dependent process, e.g. cell respiration or protein synthesis, will function any more efficiently than its least effectively supplied component. For example, the rate of a metabolic chain reaction that requires B_2 for one step, B_6 for a second, folic acid for a third, and B_{12} for a fourth will be dependent on that B vitamin that is in the shortest supply. If B_6 is the least available of the four co-enzymes, multiplying the concentrations of the other three will not accelerate or improve the overall process, which will remain dependent on the usable quantities of B_6. This is not to imply that vitamins are needed by the body in equal amounts. Not all cells require every vitamin. Some vitamins are involved in many more activities than others within a particular tissue. Some are needed in intense concentrations within a few highly specialized organs. However, supplementation that fails to include all of the vitamins, minimizes the intake of one, or exaggerates the use of any—with the possible exception of vitamin C—is apt to be futile.

- *Concentrated:* The balanced addition of vitamins to your diet in quantities equal to or exceeding U.S. RDAs will prevent the development of outright deficiency diseases. The rate and degree of compensation for prolonged sub-clinical deprivation will be proportional to the concentration of supplementation. Amounts that achieve consistent saturation will predictably yield the most complete and rapid correction of reversible tissue injury while attaining optimal metabolic function. Smaller concentrations will produce relatively slower, less certain remission and ultimate metabolic effectiveness.

Although you can reduce your vitamin requirements by eliminating processed carbohydrates, junk foods, alcohol, caffeine, additives, and preservatives from your diet and increase natural vitamin intake by relying on fresh fruits, produce, and organ meats, it is doubtful whether you can fully compensate for past deficiencies or fully meet current optimal requirements with your knife and fork. Since no one wants to take massive amounts of vitamins forever, it is probably wise to begin supplementation in concentrations designed to achieve rapid saturation without risking toxification. Maintaining safe vitamin concentrations in tissue-loading amounts should achieve appropriate compensation and optimal function within a few months. A gradual reduction in intake should follow. Your body will tell you how you feel as you reduce supplementation to appropriate maintenance levels.

● *Continuous:* Vitamins, unlike drugs, achieve their therapeutic effects slowly. Because the regeneration of cells and tissues takes time, weeks or months of comprehensive and concentrated supplementation may be necessary to compensate for deficiencies that have been acquired and sustained over many years. Improvement in your feeling of general health and well-being is apt to occur subtly, almost imperceptibly. It may produce a positive sense of greater vitality or assume the less dramatic guise of feeling less easily fatigued. Because vitamins are foods and the benefits of good nutrition are realized gradually, you may properly compare a regimen of supplementation with the training program of an athlete. Both require diligent and continuous practice if peak performance is to be achieved. Once conditioned to optimal vitamin nutrition or physical fitness, the body requires less concentrated intake or activity to maintain its improved level of function, but even reduced supplementation or exercise must be practiced consistently if physical benefits are to be permanent. However, achieving optimal vitamin intake for even a short period of time is beneficial just as attaining temporary physical fitness is of greater value than remaining forever flabby and out of shape.

● *Individualized:* Most proponents of optimum vitamin nutrition recommend individualizing your intake according to age, sex, body build, medical history, dietary habits, and other personal factors that make each of us unique. A 200-pound, 22-year-old lumberjack who needs from 3,000 to 4,000 calories to maintain his weight will, for example, require a generally higher level of supplementation than a 95-pound, 35-year-old executive secretary who keeps her size 6 figure on 1,000 calories a day.

In individualizing any program of optimal vitamin nutrition, it is essential to consider such variables as your—

• • AGE: Vitamin supplementation for infants and young children is a standard medical practice. Rely on your pediatrician for guidance, but be aware that the dietary habits a youngster establishes under your supervision during his or her formative years will profoundly affect growth and development, future health, and nutritional patterns for a lifetime. Teaching a child to eat whole, fresh foods instead of processed substitutes while emphasizing protein at the expense of carbohydrates and fats can be one of the richest legacies you may bestow on your offspring. The gift of nutritional wisdom will be put rapidly to the test during adolescence when peer pressure in favor of vitamin-poor "fast" foods holds its greatest appeal. A calorie-laden but nutritionally impoverished diet during the years following puberty is implicated in creating the biochemical conditions leading to diabetes, heart disease, arthritis, and other degenerative disorders in the third, fourth, and fifth decades of life. Because it becomes increasingly difficult to monitor an adolescent's eating habits or use of alcohol, tobacco, caffeine, and other drugs, you may be wise to encourage his or her consumption of vitamins under the direction of a nutritionally savvy physician. By the time of physical maturity at 18 or 19, regular supplementation may be as important a personal habit as routine practices of hygiene, contraception, and prophylaxis.

Because adulthood cannot be neatly subdivided into such predictable phases as infancy, childhood, and adolescence, attempts to categorize the mature years must be artificial and thought of only in the broadest of terms:

AGES 19–35: For most people this is a time of peak

physical conditioning and activity when the body tends to be most resilient, often withstanding repeated insult without betraying more than temporary symptoms of abuse. It is also a time of considerable physiological and emotional stress when women normally bear their children and men struggle to establish a career and provide for their families. Failure to rest sufficiently, exercise adequately, and/or eat properly are typical transitional problems of early maturity that may become habituated with repetition and be compounded by recourse to alcohol, prescription medications, and other socially approved "crutches" or panaceas in our overwrought society. Although injury is apt to be imperceptible, the continuous physical and emotional stress of these years can create the kinds of metabolic strain that lead to most sub-clinical vitamin deficiencies and the subsequent degeneration of body tissue.

AGES 36–50: In the ordinary course of human events this period is one of peak productivity that secures social stability and the attainment of economic prosperity. The efforts of a lifetime are either supported or suborned by our physical well-being during these all-important years. Although maximum body fitness is past, the quality of fiber and sinew can remain vigorous and resilient as a result of intelligent care and maintenance. Bodily assaults that could earlier be absorbed without apparent ill effect now produce increasingly obvious and harmful injury. If cumulative abuse has been extravagant, premature mortality or permanently crippling disease may be the result. Attention to the fundamental principles of good health is critical if vitality is to be retained throughout a lifetime. For most of us the body still possesses sufficient elasticity during these years to either correct or arrest the ravages of prior maltreatment.

AGE 51+: Although our contemporary society and environment raise numerous obstacles to longevity, there are few biological reasons why the human body can't survive for eighty years or more. Barring accidents and excessive physical abuse, we are designed to live vigorous and active lives for eight decades or more with only a brief period of decay and senescence preceding death. Maintenance of optimal vitamin nutrition is crucial to the quality of life during these golden years. After thousands of cell replications, which began before birth, errors in protein metabolism invariably occur, with the result that our tissues produce fewer functional enzyme molecules than when we were younger. Making certain that ample supplies of vitamin co-enzymes are available to the reduced number of appropriate protein molecules is essential. Normal vitamin supplies may be subverted if apathy or boredom—sometimes typical of aging— produces indifference to good nutrition. Because physical activity and our need for calories tend to lessen with advancing years, reduced food intake may create nutritional deprivation since vitamin requirements tend to remain constant or increase with age. Dental difficulties, lessened digestive function, and absorptive disorders may impair our ability to obtain dietary vitamins from the food we eat, while chronic or infectious disease, acquired vitamin dependence, or metabolic inefficiency actually elevate our need for these essential nutrients.

- SEX: Although women live longer and are generally less susceptible to devastating degenerative diseases than men, they are more vulnerable to minor ailments and complaints than their male counterparts. Close to 70 percent of all medical appointments and more than 60 percent of prorated employee absences involve women. Although this disparity between the sexes may be partly attributed to social and psychological factors in our male-dominated society, sub-clinical vitamin deficiencies related to female biochemistry may be a hidden but vital cause for such phenomena. During the reproductive years, which may extend from 15 to 50, a woman's body undergoes continuous cyclic stress resulting from the metabolic and hormonal effort required to produce a mature egg, or ovum. The periodic menstrual flow that accompanies the ejection of an unfertilized egg reduces her blood supply and often creates symptoms of anemia associated with the loss of iron from the body. Replenishment of lost blood requires increased vitamin metabolism, as does the formation of the next mature egg. Failure to supply additional vitamins to her system during ovulation and menstruation subjects a woman to periodic sub-clinical deficiencies that may continue for thirty years or more and permanently elevate her need for the various vitamins.

If fertilization occurs, a woman's body experiences profound physiological changes that greatly increase her metabolic and nutritional requirements. Pregnancy demands that a mother-to-be not only support her own heightened metabolism but supply all of the nutritional raw materials essential to the developing fetus. If her diet cannot provide the requisite amino acids, simple sugars, fatty acids, vitamins, and minerals, her body will cannibalize its own cells and tissues to release the necessary nutrients for fetal use. Because adequate caloric intake is not an endemic problem in this country, most women can supply their unborn with ample quantities of proteins, carbohydrates, and fats. However, the prevalence of marginal vitamin nutrition among women of child-bearing age may well account for the alarming rate of miscarriages, stillbirths, underweight babies, and infant mortality typical of America today. Lack of sufficient vitamin supplies may cause the metabolic rejection of a developing fetus or impair its normal growth and development. Although vitamin supplementation during pregnancy is universally practiced in most advanced nations, such supportive measures are only inconsistently applied here. Even if prescribed during pregnancy, vitamin therapy often ends with parturition—although the nursing, or lactating, female continues to draw heavily on her dietary resources or vitamin stores in supplying milk to her suckling infant. The current obstetric and gynecologic practice of using diuretic drugs to reduce the accumulation of tissue fluid during gestation, lactation, or menstruation exacerbates female vitamin deficiencies since the flushing action of such medications eliminates many water-soluble vitamins from the body.

Although the widespread use of oral contraceptives has prevented many unwanted pregnancies, the benefits of "the Pill" may be nullified by the side effects and adverse reactions experienced by many women. The continued use of estrogen contraceptives after 30 years of age is closely linked to the premature occurrence of heart and circulatory disorders. Evidence that the contraceptive function of estrogen requires greatly increased quantities of vitamins—particularly those of the B complex—is highly suggestive, and vitamin supplementation for women taking the Pill is gaining general medical acceptance.

For biochemical reasons that are not fully understood, women tend to lose their comparative immunity from degenerative diseases following menopause. The incidence of heart attacks, arthritis, diabetes, and other lethal or disabling disorders tends to be equal for both males and females over 45 years of age. Although men do not suffer from natural physiological stresses equivalent to those of the mature female, their larger body weight, typically greater physical activity, and macho tendencies to overlook bodily discomforts often create a considerable gap between their optimum vitamin needs and actual vitamin input. On balance, while a female may be smaller and lighter than male counterparts, her reproductive years— with the pressures of menstruation, pregnancy, lactation, and/or oral contraception—may make her need for vitamins greater on a pound-for-pound basis than a man's. Such gender-based considerations must be taken into account when planning any program of vitamin supplementation.

• • BODY BUILD: Although the "average" body is composed of about 50 trillion cells, there is a significant difference in cell number between the individual weighing-in at the usual adult minimum of 75 pounds and the individual who tips the scale at the typical maximum of 300 pounds. The fourfold difference between the two extremes in avoirdupois does not represent a corresponding difference in number of body cells. The heavier individual is apt to possess greater height, more massive bone structure, and larger deposits of non-cellular fat than a less hefty counterpart. While greater body weight and number of body cells seem to demand a proportionately more concentrated supply of vitamins for optimal function, the correlation is not absolute. The ratio between flesh and bone is important. Among people of the same weight, those of greater height and broader skeletal structure usually require fewer vitamins than those who are comparatively more compact, adipose, or muscular.

In attempting to estimate your vitamin needs from the OPA recommendations, remember that stated values are only approximate. Two people with a difference in weight of 40 pounds and a variation in height of 10 inches may potentially achieve tissue saturation at the same level of vitamin intake. Having found your appropriate height/weight category and evaluated your particular body build, select your level of supplementation within the stated range of concentration on the basis of such individualized factors as age, sex, particular lifestyle, and medical history.

• • PERSONAL FACTORS: The most important determinants of our optimum vitamin requirements are often the most elusive and difficult to define. No instrument can now measure our inherited nutritional needs. Precisely evaluating past medical and dietary history is tricky. To know, for example, to what degree the positive personal advantages of a lifetime without cigarette smoking, the consumption of alcohol, or the use of drugs may have offset the socially enforced negatives of living in an industrialized and polluted urban environment is beyond the reach of physicians, biochemists, and laymen. Our best clues probably involve our relative sense of physical well-being. Ready susceptibility to colds and other infections, vulnerability to fatigue, lack of vigor, and loss of physical suppleness are general indicators that the composite value of all the factors in our lives—past and present—has produced a state of health that is far from optimum.

Because there are so many variables that have made us what we are today, it is probably best to take an experimental approach to supplementation. By consuming mid-range values for *all* of the various vitamins over a period of at least four to six weeks, you can begin to assess their nutritional relevance for you. Increased stamina, lessened fatigue, and greater resistance to minor ailments are typical body signals that indicate sub-clinical vitamin deficiencies have been a limiting factor to your health and that their correction is in progress. After a period of three to four months of supplementation you may reduce your intake of all the vitamins in stages until you find the maintenance levels appropriate for your unique body chemistry. Should you experience any physical setbacks following decreased ingestion, it is wise to return to previously effective levels of consumption.

If after one month you can detect no improvement in your general state of well-being, it is reasonable to increase your vitamin intake to higher levels *within your supplement category*. If after an additional six to eight weeks you perceive no physical benefits from supplementation, then it is logical to gradually cut your consumption to U.S. RDA values. Factors other than vitamin deprivation are probably impeding your health, and until they are corrected, continued supplementation beyond that necessary to prevent deficiency disorders is apt to prove both costly and futile.

● *Categorized:* Before beginning a program of vitamin supplementation, it is important to understand the distinctions among the various sources and classes of these compounds. Whether consumed with our knives and forks or in tablet, liquid, or capsule form, the function of vitamins is purely nutritional. Dietary supplies of these substances are uncertain because modern handling, processing, and preparation rob most foods of their intrinsic vitamin content. Such traditional sources are also unreliable since menu choices tend to change dramatically from day to day. Unless you regularly consume large quantities of whole and unprocessed foods, it is probably wise to consider the vitamins you derive from your diet as a nutritional dividend while planning to obtain your OPA quantities from the supplement product(s) you choose.

Although it is essential that all of the recognized vitamins be taken both intensively and persistently to achieve optimum nutrition, consideration of the unique characteristics of their various forms and different varieties is essential to intelligent supplementation. The categories include—

- • THE FAT-SOLUBLE VITAMINS: Because the body can retain quantities of A, D, E, and K that it does not immediately need, there is a remote possibility that extravagant intake of these nutrients may overload storage tissue and produce unpleasant side effects, e.g. headache or nausea, that disappear when supplementation ceases. The maximum OPA quantities listed here are at concentration levels that are no more than 1/20th, or 5 percent, of those daily amounts that may exceed your body's tolerance. To ensure absolute safety you may independently control your ingestion of A, D, and E by taking a specific product that contains only fat-soluble vitamins while relying on another for the balance of your supplementation. Consuming small quantities of fats or oils (normally found in meats, salad dressings, etc.) along with these vitamins will help guarantee their proper absorption across the intestinal wall.

- • THE ESSENTIAL B-COMPLEX VITAMINS: These synergistic nutrients must be consumed together in balanced quantities to be effective. They include thiamin (B_1), riboflavin (B_2), niacin (B_3), B_6, B_{12}, folic acid, biotin, and pantothenic acid. Because these vitamins are rapidly excreted from the body, you can maintain most consistent and continuous body concentrations by dividing your daily allowance into two or three equal portions and spacing their intake at appropriate eight- or twelve-hour intervals.

- • THE CONTESTED VITAMINS: These water-soluble compounds include inositol, para aminobenzoic acid (PABA), pangamate (B_{15}), and the bioflavonoids. Until their biochemical status is clarified, you may consider their use as optional. Their inclusion on the OPA chart (pages 154–155) is at concentrations recommended by those nutritionists, physicians, and chemists who recognize their legitimate function as vitamins. No one denies their normal occurrence in the body, and consumption at these levels is safe but of uncertain effectiveness.

• • VITAMIN C: This water-soluble vitamin must be considered separately from all others because of the controversy surrounding its evolutionary significance, biochemical function, and potential human use. Eminent opinion suggests that man and his close relations lost their capacity to synthesize this essential nutrient as the result of a favorable mutation that occurred among our common ancestors millions of years ago. It is believed that these distant forebears once obtained from 4 to 5 grams of the vitamin from their normal daily diet as do our great ape and primate relatives today. Loss of the synthesizing capacity—when dietary supplies were abundant—arguably made cellular room for other more valuable and advantageous biochemical mechanisms to evolve. A contrasting opinion supports the idea that man once consumed far larger quantities of C than he does now but suggests that failure of the synthetic ability was a ghastly rather than favorable genetic mistake. It argues that a majority of man's ills in modern times may be traced to his enormous and unfulfilled need for the nutrient and that we should all consume from 3 to 5 grams of C per day to achieve optimum metabolic function and thereby protect ourselves from infectious and degenerative illness.[2]

Controversy concerning the ingestion of large quantities of C to prevent or combat the symptoms
(Text continued on page 156)

2. If these arguments prove correct, we may have been unwittingly interfering with normal evolutionary processes by favoring the selection and survival of men who have abnormally low metabolic requirements —not only for C, but for all of the vitamins.

Recommended Optimum Personal

	Weight (±20 lbs)	Height (±5″)	Fat-Soluble Vitamins			Water-Soluble Vitamins (Essential)		
			Vitamin A (IU)	Vitamin D (IU)	Vitamin E (IU)	Vitamin C (mg)	Folic Acid — (mcg)	Thiamin B₁ (mg)
Males								
Age: 19–35	147	69						
Lower limit			5,000	400	100	1,000	500	50
Upper limit			10,000	600	200	2,000	1,000	150
Age: 36–50	154	69						
Lower limit			5,000	400	200	1,000	500	100
Upper limit			10,000	600	400	3,000	1,000	150
Age: 51+	154	69						
Lower limit			10,000	400	400	2,000	500	100
Upper limit			15,000	600	600	4,000	1,000	200
Females								
Age: 19–35	128	65						
Lower limit			5,000	400	100	1,000	500	50
Upper limit			10,000	600	200	2,000	1,000	150
Age: 36–50	128	65						
Lower limit			7,000	400	100	1,000	500	100
Upper limit			12,000	600	300	3,000	1,000	150
Age: 51+	128	65						
Lower limit			10,000	600	400	2,000	500	100
Upper limit			15,000	800	600	4,000	1,000	200

NOTES

a. You may not require vitamin A supplementation if you regularly consume organ meats, lamb chops, or sweet potatoes—all of which contain high concentrations of the compound or its precursor, carotene. A typical 4- to 6-ounce serving of liver alone will provide you with from 60,000 to 80,000 IU of A.

b. Four 8-ounce glasses of fortified milk will meet your OPA requirements for D. Although few foods besides fish oils contain natural and significant quantities of the vitamin, frequent exposure to tanning rays from the sun will stimulate skin production of ample quantities of D. Be sure to consider these factors in planning your supplementation.

Allowances (OPAs) for Vitamins

Essential Water-Soluble Vitamins cont'd						Water-Soluble Vitamins (Contested)			
Riboflavin B$_2$ (mg)	Niacin B$_3$ (mg)	Vitamin B$_6$ (mg)	Vitamin B$_{12}$ (mcg)	Biotin — (mcg)	Pantothenic Acid — (mg)	Inositol (mg)	PABA (mg)	Pangamate (mg)	Bioflavonoids (mg)
50	100	50	50	50	100	100	50	25	50
150	300	150	150	150	200	200	150	75	100
100	100	100	100	100	100	100	100	25	50
150	300	200	150	150	200	200	150	75	100
100	200	100	100	100	100	100	100	25	50
200	400	200	200	200	300	300	200	50	100
50	100	100	50	50	100	100	50	25	50
150	300	200	150	150	200	200	150	75	100
100	100	200	100	100	100	100	100	25	50
150	300	300	150	150	200	200	150	75	100
100	200	100	100	100	100	100	100	25	50
200	400	200	200	200	300	300	200	50	100

c. Even though the FDA rates vitamin E as virtually non-toxic (because little of the compound can be stored by body tissues), it may elevate blood pressure and is potentially hazardous—when used indiscriminately—for those suffering from hypertension or heart disease. Do not take more than 200 IU a day without medical assurance that your blood pressure is normal and that you are free from disease symptoms.

d. Vitamin K deficiency is extremely rare. Its correction requires the close supervision of a knowledgeable physician. Avoid any supplement product that contains the compound.

e. Unlike most of its B-complex counterparts, large quantities of choline are synthesized by the body from raw foodstuffs. It is probably unnecessary to supplement your diet with the vitamin, but it is safe to do so since the substance is both water soluble and non-toxic.

f. Because deficiencies of different B-complex compounds cause or aggravate different forms of anemia, all of the essential B vitamins must be taken together in balanced quantities. An excess of folic acid may, for example, mask the symptoms of B_{12} deprivation.

g. IU = International Units; mg = milligrams; mcg = micrograms.

h. For greatest flexibility, you may wish to choose three separate supplement products—one containing the fat-soluble vitamins, another with the water-soluble forms, and a third with vitamin C alone.

i. Be certain to refer to Appendix D, "Personal Vitamin Planner," for help in creating your individual OPA program.

• • VITAMIN C: *(Continued from page 153)*

of the common cold has obscured the fundamental and proper nutritional uses of the compound. Proponents of vitamin C therapy contend that at the first signs of an impending infection intake should be stepped-up to as much as 10 to 15 grams per day. Although there has been much public and professional discussion about the vitamin, there has been little rigorous testing to support or deny its efficacy in either preventing or curing a cold. Critics can cite numerous but inconclusive studies that indicate no difference in the incidence of the disorder between those people who used no supplemental C and others who consumed from 1 to 5 grams of the vitamin per day. Advocates often refer to the same studies but draw very different conclusions from the same data. They can demonstrate that while there were no statistically significant differences in the occurrence of colds, those who supplemented their diets with C suffered far milder symptoms, required up to 50 percent fewer medical visits, and lost only a fraction of the workdays of their unprotected counterparts. Indeed, the best current evidence suggests that vitamin C will probably not prevent your cold or other infectious disorder but will help improve your overall stamina, body function, and general good health. For you to use C—or any other vitamin—for the *treatment* of disease symptoms violates the fundamental precepts of supplementation and is of questionable wisdom. You must be the judge.

6

Vitamins: Their Uses and Abuses

The cautious seldom err.
— CONFUCIUS

THE PERSONAL USE OF VITAMINS

Because few, if any, of us have led or will ever lead lives in the best of all possible biochemical worlds, any positive step we take to compensate for past assaults or future transgressions against our physical selves must be counted among the personal treasures we lay-up before entering the kingdom of heaven or its alternative. By enriching our daily diets with essential vitamins we assist the body in its lifelong struggle for survival and help protect the flesh against the inevitable onslaught of the aging process. To understand the nature and extent of the rewards we may reasonably anticipate from supplementation and to appreciate their very real limitations is of critical importance. We may expect that the intelligent use of vitamins will—

- help improve our general level of health.

- help lessen, defer, or prevent the injury of infectious

and degenerative disease, the debilitation of aging, and the occurrence of premature mortality.

- help correct past abuses of the body due to poor nutrition; excessive fatigue; tension; the consumption of alcohol, nicotine, drugs, or other personal poisons; the metabolic stresses of acute illness, childbearing, or chronic disease; and the strain of life in our contemporary and polluted environment.

- be of definite biological benefit without any certainty of what the ultimate and *specific* advantages will be. The symptoms of both clinical and sub-clinical deficiencies are rarely well defined and are often confusing. Dry and itching skin may, for example, be a product of too little vitamin A in one person but have quite a different origin in another.

Although the biochemical changes that result from deprivation are frequently predictable from known molecular functions of the various vitamins, outward and visible symptoms may or may not reveal their relationship to the impaired internal reactions that cause them. Most deficiencies are manifested by a general reduction in metabolic effectiveness and produce symptoms unique to us as individuals. It is only after intensive, balanced, and persistent use that some of the specific, personal values of supplementation become apparent. To associate particular nutritional deficiencies with individual symptoms or illness and to attempt their treatment with vitamins—as many enthusiasts suggest—is reckless. With the possible exception of C and the common cold, there are no legitimate therapeutic uses for vitamins without benefit of a knowledgeable medical practitioner. It is wise to take supplements to improve our health, but foolish not to see a doctor at the first signs or symptoms of disease.

THE MEDICAL USES OF VITAMINS

Physicians routinely prescribe vitamins in varying amounts for infants, children, and the aged. They often recommend supplementation for pregnant women, nursing mothers, and those with inadequate or specialized diets that are intended to promote weight loss, conform to religious doctrine, or fulfill exceptional needs due to vigorous exercise, severe illness, or surgery. Individuals suffering from genetic abnormalities, impaired digestive and absorptive function, or acute debilitation are likely to need vitamins by injection to sustain their lives.

Because individual vitamins are so intimately and critically involved with the tissues and organs prone to disorder, increasing numbers of medical practitioners are using massive supplementation to prevent, cure, or relieve many of the more refractory diseases that plague our age. It is biochemically logical that the metabolic malfunction and disequilibrium typical of many disorders may respond to very concentrated levels of vitamin infusion. Although the possibility that such nutritional therapy may ease human suffering is intriguing, *its use must remain in the exclusive domain of the trained medical professional.*[1]

SCHIZOPHRENIA AND OTHER NERVOUS SYSTEM DISORDERS

When Sigmund Freud first expounded his theory of personality during the closing years of the last century, he clearly expressed his belief that both the normal and aberrative functions of the human mind would one day be explained in terms of brain and body chemistry. He offered his psychoanalytic techniques for the treatment of mental disorders and personality dysfunctions as immediate therapy to relieve a patient's distress until that time when such problems could be diagnosed and cured by manipulation of brain and nervous system metabolism. Although Freud's methods and those of both his orthodox and renegade disciples have had profound effect on western civilization, their applicability and usefulness in treating mental illness have been limited. The "talk and reflect" approach of the various psychoanalytic schools has un-

---

1. See Appendix A for access to directories of medically qualified, nutritionally oriented physicians, dentists, and other health professionals.

doubted benefits for those suffering from the milder forms of anxiety, depression, and similar neuroses. It has little effect on such severe disorders as schizophrenia, acute paranoia, and other psychoses that usually require hospitalization.

Although the medical establishment has traditionally ignored minor mental and emotional complaints while coping with acute insanity by anesthetizing the sufferer into somnolence, recent biochemical research has begun to produce the kinds of metabolic understanding that may fulfill Freud's original prophecy. Significant numbers of previously incurable schizophrenics, manic-depressives, and autistic children have achieved an often complete remission of symptoms through exacting nutritional therapy and specific vitamin supplementation. Treatment includes removing all food additives, preservatives, and other potentially irritating compounds, such as caffeine, from the diet. Eliminating sugar and reducing starch intake while emphasizing the frequent consumption of protein apparently helps stabilize metabolism, correct chemical imbalances, and prevent the physiological fluctuations that trigger uncontrolled emotional outbursts. Critical to this form of therapy is the use of massive quantities of those B-complex vitamins, C, and E essential to the function of all nerve cells. Niacin, or B_3, alone, in 3- to 15-*gram* quantities often produces a startling reversal of aberrant behaviors. That a percentage of any population should have an abnormally high and unfulfilled need for a vitamin is predictable. That symptoms of psychosis are typical of the clinical B_3 depletion disease (pellagra) suggests that many of our mentally ill may be so, *not* because of traumatic emotional experiences in childhood, but as a result of a severe nutritional deficiency or metabolic imbalance that can be corrected by careful attention to the sufferer's unique body chemistry.

HEART AND OTHER CIRCULATORY DISORDERS

Biological failure of the human heart and circulatory system accounts for more than half the deaths in this country. Breakdown of the cardiac pump and its conduits usually occurs long before the collapse of other body tissue —yet the heart and blood vessels are far more resistant to infection than other less vulnerable organs and systems. Although genetic predisposition affects susceptibility, coronary and circulatory disorders are not strictly inherited as are eye color or blood type. Like most forms of diabetes, arthritis, and possibly cancer, heart and related diseases seem to be metabolic disorders that result from conflict between our inherited biochemistry and the environmental conditions in which it must function. The food we eat, air we breathe, water we drink, and our idiosyncratic personal habits evidently conspire to damage our cardiac tissue and circulatory system. Although modern medicine has invented brilliant devices to replace defective valves, worn-out vessels, and—potentially—the whole heart, while developing powerful drugs that thin the blood and reduce the pressure of its flow, all of these techniques aim only at relieving symptoms. They do not attack and eliminate the causes that lead to degeneration and deterioration in the first place.

Although cigarette smoking is a prime culprit in robbing us of our coronary health and circulatory vitality, many people who have never used tobacco suffer from cerebral hemorrhages, cardio-vascular accidents, and arteriosclerosis. It is the nature and quality of our diets that is increasingly implicated in the widespread incidence of such cardiac diseases.[2] A lifetime of eating nutritionally impoverished processed foods rich in refined starches, sugars, and fats can cause profound changes in heart and circulatory tissue that lead to premature deterioration and demise. Because vegetarians do not necessarily escape the lethal build-up of cholesterol in their blood vessels, simply avoiding animal fats is no cardiac cure-all.

A number of research physicians and practitioners have had striking successes in preventing the recurrence

---

2. Recent studies indicate that inadequate exercise is a less significant factor in promoting circulatory ill health than generally thought. Although jogging is of benefit to body tone and suppleness, it does not seem to lower the rate of heart attacks for either men or women.

of heart attacks and circulatory accidents by paying close attention to the logic of a patient's individual metabolic history. They often prescribe massive doses of thiamin, or B_1—reasoning that a lifetime of excessive carbohydrate consumption probably elevates metabolic requirements for the vitamin on a permanent basis, even after excessive ingestion has been greatly reduced. Similar amounts of vitamin E are included in treatment to ensure proper metabolism of the polyunsaturated oils that replace animal fats in the cardiac's dietary regimen. Use of this fat-soluble vitamin demonstrably reduces the pain of *angina pectoris* and *intermittent claudication,* the cramping of leg muscles that makes walking difficult for many individuals with poor circulation. Because high-protein diets can be correlated with a low incidence of heart disease, supplementation with generous amounts of B_2 and B_6 is a logical adjunct to nutritional therapy.

Although the prevention or treatment of heart and circulatory disorders involves many variables, massive doses of appropriate vitamins may well be a key—if often overlooked—factor to success.

ARTHRITIS, CANCER, AND OTHER CONTEMPORARY DISEASES

Low concentrations of pantothenic acid are often noted in the adrenal cortex of people suffering from rheumatoid and other forms of arthritis. Because this glandular tissue produces the body's supply of steroid hormones that regulates the mineralization of bone, any undersecretion of these compounds may be associated with developing joint disease and can potentially be corrected through supplementation.

Laetrile, a vitaminlike compound extracted from apricots, is a highly controversial substance that has been used to relieve suffering among the victims of terminal cancer. Although recognized as a legitimate therapy in more than twenty nations, its use in this country has been strongly opposed by the FDA and medical establishment.

Whether the substance can disrupt the reproductive processes of malignant cells—as suggested by foreign medical reports—remains to be seen.

Unfortunately, the furor over Laetrile tends to obscure more promising uses of vitamins in protecting the body against cancer. Because vitamin C prevents the breakdown of fertilizer nitrates and food-additive nitrites into carcinogenic nitrosamines, it certainly helps thwart malignancy. Vitamins A and E may have the same kind of immunizing function, while it is within the realm of possibility that the stimulus needed to convert ordinary cells into cancerous aberrants may come from prolonged vitamin starvation.

Although the medical literature is increasingly rife with reports that virtually all human illness—from allergies and asthma to zymogenosis and zymotic disease—responds to treatment with various vitamin supplements, few cures, if any, have been confirmed beyond all reasonable doubt. While vitamins in theory have tremendous medical potential, their effectiveness in practice has yet to be proved.

THE MISUSE OF VITAMIN SUPPLEMENTS

Because all of the various vitamins are native to human tissue and can be tolerated in very large quantities without side effect or adverse reaction, their use in supplementation poses little threat to the body's integrity and well-being. Excessive consumption of any other ordinary food—protein, carbohydrate, fat, or mineral—produces more serious chemical imbalances than overload quantities of vitamins, which are simply stored or excreted in amounts exceeding those the body can use. Given this biochemical amiability and the promise of generous rewards with a minimum of risk, many people develop an enthusiasm for vitamins that overrides their usual mother wit and native caution. Although vitamins offer none of the potential for habituation, dependence, or injury associated with drugs, their uncritical and inappropriate use can be harmful. For anyone about to begin a regimen of supplementation, the following caveats and concerns are of importance.

- Attempting to treat any personal symptoms of illness (other than those of the common cold) with vitamins is folly. Many prominent nutritional extremists and "experts" have died disconcertingly young because they did not seek medical help when they needed it. Get your physician's advice if you suspect ill health. Use vitamins to prevent it.

- Nothing could be more foolhardy for the layman than to undertake self-diagnosis of single or multiple vitamin deficiencies. Most medical doctors cannot identify those vitamins—particularly those of the B complex—that are in short supply, and even sophisticated biochemical techniques are not entirely reliable detectors of deficiency. To exaggerate your intake of one or a few vitamins—except C—flies in the face of sound reason and good judgement.

- Do not begin a program of supplementation without consulting your physician if you are taking medications he has prescribed or suffer from any chronic or acute disorder. Vitamin C magnifies the effects of oral insulins, and a diabetic's normal intake of the hormone may produce severe shock in the presence of C. Because of their effect on cholesterol metabolism, the ingestion of niacin, pantothenic acid, or E may interfere with or exaggerate the action of anticoagulant or antihypertensive medications used by cardiac patients. Since vitamins naturally affect the chemistry of tissue fluids, they often alter the results of routine laboratory tests. Technicians and physicians should be informed of your supplementation before analyzing blood or urine samples.

- Be certain to stop supplementation at the first sign of any negative or untoward symptom. Mild digestive upset is not uncommon when beginning intake. Disturbance is often the result of negative response to the binders and fillers used in formulating a supplement product. Switching brands or taking your vitamins along with food will probably correct such difficulty.

● Be certain to avoid all nutritional fads and fetishes. Media reporters, their editorial superiors, and the manufacturers of supplement products know that the periodic "discovery" of miraculous and hitherto unknown vitamin properties can sell many newspapers, while galvanizing the public into an orgy of uncritical supplement buying and usage. The recent rage for E (because of its reputed ability to renew sexual vigor) had its origins in the well-documented fact that the gonads of the rat require the vitamin to achieve maturity and maintain full function. What is libidinously true for a rodent has no comparable relevance for man. While nutritional hype may be good for the national economy, it is of questionable personal benefit for your body. Avoid its blandishments whenever you can.

● Do not put all of your nutritional eggs in one basket. Relying on vitamins alone for good health is absurd. Your chances for physical well-being depend on many factors. Ample rest, appropriate exercise, and an intelligent diet are a few of the imperatives. Supplementation can only support and reinforce sound health practices. It cannot bestow immunity on a body that continues to be metabolically maltreated and physically abused.

7

How to Select a Vitamin Supplement

When you buy, use your eyes and your mind, not your ears.

— CZECH PROVERB

The compounding, marketing, promotion, and sale of vitamin supplements is a billion-dollar business. Most of the major pharmaceutical houses compete with one another and a host of independent producers, health food companies, and mail order houses for your almighty dollar. On entering the typical drugstore or health food shop, you are apt to confront a dazzling array of products. As many as two hundred different varieties of single vitamin, multivitamin, and multivitamin/multimineral supplements may be on display. Each is cleverly packaged in the best tradition of Madison Avenue. Labels—except for single-ingredient products—often require a magnifying glass for legibility and a medical dictionary for comprehension. Confusion, bewilderment, anger, frustration, and embarrassment are frequent reactions to such encounters with the vitamin marketplace. Many supplement formulations are irrational, and so are most attempts to evaluate a whole range of products in a few minutes spent at the display rack. You *can* make intelligent product choices that do fulfill your needs, assure you of quality, but don't drain your pocketbook. Your shopping must begin before you arrive at the vitamin counter.

NATURAL (ORGANIC) VS. MANUFACTURED (SYNTHETIC) VITAMINS

Considerable time, money, and talk are annually expended to convince us that vitamins from "natural" sources are superior to those of "industrial" origin. The popularity of the good earth, back-to-nature movement and its positive goals are often cynically exploited when applied to vitamin promotions. The claim that a supplement is "natural" or "organic" aims at our approval of the cleaner-than-clean, Walden Pond freshness so cunningly employed by cigarette manufacturers. In truth, the word "natural" is a shorthand for "extracted from natural sources," i.e. derived from plant or animal material. The extraction process itself may require use of the very same harsh solvents, high heat, and pressure that, by implication, are so assiduously avoided in compounding a product. Often the amount of a given vitamin extracted from such natural resources by highly artificial means is far below essential strength, and the required concentrations must be met by the addition of manufactured vitamins. Vitamin C from the fleshy base, or hip, of a rose is the most conspicuous example. To contain sufficient quantities of pure rose hip C, a supplement would be as big as a hen's egg. To overcome this inconvenience, manufacturers most often compound a product with 5 percent of the "natural" vitamin along with 95 percent from so-called synthetic sources. That the resulting supplement is sold as Rose Hip Vitamin C, usually at inflated prices, is a rip-off.[1]

---

1. Claims that vitamins have been derived from "organic" or "natural" sources are not always irrelevant or fraudulent. When vitamins can be extracted from living tissue in sufficient quantity without excessive chemical torture, they may provide additional nutrients or improve absorbability, e.g. the fat-soluble A, D, and E in fish oils, or vitamin C in combination with its chemical allies—the bioflavonoids (rutin, hesperidin, acerola, etc.). However, the obvious gimmick has been so broadly abused that the bad apples have largely spoiled the barrel and caution is advisable.

When a supplement is described as "organic," you may suffer from a similar abuse in terminology and cost. Any molecule containing carbon, hydrogen, and oxygen is properly described as organic. Coal tar, plastics, and petroleum products all qualify but hardly fulfill the expectations aroused. Organically grown fruits and vegetables are ones raised without the use of commercial fertilizers, pesticides, and sprays. By a verbal sleight-of-hand, "organic" has been employed by some vitamin producers in a manner not too different from that used by sanitationmen when they style themselves "ecological engineers." When applied to a vitamin supplement, the term "organic" simply means that a portion of the product has been extracted from plant or animal tissue. It is rare for a label to indicate what proportion of a vitamin comes from such tissue or what extraction processes were employed in its retrieval.

Synthetic vitamins are as poorly named as their "natural" or "organic" counterparts. Because most people associate the term with artificiality and inferiority, it is easy to exploit your distaste for the "synthetic." Such vitamins are more accurately described as "synthesized"—often by processes employing such "natural" factories as yeasts, molds, and other micro-organisms. Contrary to the claims of extreme health food enthusiasts, who tout the absolute and unvarying superiority of "organic" or "natural" vitamins, there is no known biochemical difference between a *pure* vitamin derived from living tissue and one synthesized from scratch.

VITAMIN SUPPLEMENTATION WITH ENRICHED, FORTIFIED, OR VITAMINIZED FOODS

Making a virtue of nutritionally suspect processed foods, which must by law be enriched with vitamins, is a cynical but widespread practice among the giants of the American food industry. Each morning millions breakfast with a bowl of cold, nutritionally emasculated, puffed, flaked, cracked, or tortured slush. Beguiled by one of advertising's most effective and insidious ad campaigns, a vast portion of the populace is seduced into believing they are following good health practices by swallowing their *total* Federally dictated U.S. RDAs at one sitting. This form of supplementation is probably the most widely practiced and least beneficial of all vitamin regimens.

Attempts to fortify common foods with vitamins meagerly supplied by the typical diet are well intentioned but of questionable value. Unless fresh fish is a common item on your bill of fare, you are apt to get only marginal supplies of vitamin D with your knife and fork. Recognizing that long winter months without contact between skin and sun can deplete even generous stores of D, local health authorities often order that milk be fortified with the vitamin. The ultraviolet radiation that converts Elsie's cholesterol to D also destroys members of the B complex. Robbing Peter to pay Paul by supplying one vitamin at the expense of others is a foolhardy nutritional economy.

A similar but more intelligent benevolence is at work as various regulatory agencies have tried to achieve standardization among foods subject to wide seasonal fluctuations in vitamin content. Unfortunately, attempts to maintain consistent concentrations of A and E in milk or C in orange juice have proved abortive as opposing food industry lobbies have successfully quashed any heresy that threatens to add to their production costs. A more sinister and cynical agribusiness ploy has exploited the public's concern with vitamin impoverishment and desire for food supplementation. Restoring a few of the cheaper vitamins to such nutritionally devastated products as instant mashed potatoes and proclaiming it a dietary dividend is a nutritional travesty. Even more abhorrent is the indiscriminate vitaminization of the candy, cupcakes, and other sweet subversives principally marketed for children. The mind boggles at the thought of an unsuspecting mother imagining that such supplementation will mitigate the nutritional ravages of junk food. In the face of Madison Avenue's hidden and not-so-hidden persuaders, such deceptions gain widespread acceptance. They have already convinced far too many that vitamin-hyped products fulfill the dietary needs of any and all true-blue, red-blooded Americans.

VITAMIN SUPPLEMENTATION WITH "ORGANICALLY GROWN" FOODS

The back-to-the-earth movement of the 1960s and 70s stimulated a major effort among numbers of farmers and émigré city folk to raise food crops and animal herds without enriched feeds, or commercial fertilizers, insecticides, pesticides, and other chemical interferents. Relying solely on manure for soil enrichment[2] and nineteenth-century recipes for insect and pest control, most—*but not all*—of the experiments proved biologically unsound and economically disastrous. The widespread use of chemical sprays during this century has resulted in the selection and survival of highly resistant strains of microbe, insect, and rodent, which easily decimate chemically unprotected plants and animals.

Routine chemical analysis all too frequently reveals that claimed "organically grown" fruits and vegetables contain even higher concentrations of insecticides, chemical fertilizers, and growth hormones than those raised by conventional methods. Reasons for such contamination may reflect a conscious intent to defraud, unintentional sullying, or a frantic effort to save a crop threatened with imminent extinction.

Although genuine organically grown meat and produce are available in limited quantities, demand far outstrips supply. You are wise to verify the origin of organically grown foodstuffs by dealing only with a supplier you know and trust. The nutritional rewards can be enormous.

---

2. In areas where soil is lacking essential minerals, the use of animal waste as fertilizer perpetuates the deficiency state. Feeding on grass and fodder grown on mineral-depleted soil results in manure that reflects the animal's impoverished diet.

VITAMIN SUPPLEMENTATION WITH TABLETS, CAPSULES, LIQUIDS, DROPS, OR CRYSTALS

Because they are immune to the vagaries of farming methods or climate and escape the destructive influences of processing, storage, and cooking, food supplements offer you the most reliable and efficient means for obtaining known quantities of essential vitamins. Their formulation in tablets, capsules, liquids, drops, or crystals mimics the delivery forms of most drugs. Such similarity unfortunately tends to confuse vitamins, which are foods, with medications, which are powerful substances generally alien to the body. The emulation is necessary since such fabrication maximally protects both vitamins and drugs from injury in the digestive tract.

BINDERS AND FILLERS

Many people who begin taking vitamin supplements in pill or capsule form experience unpleasant digestive side effects. Assuming that the vitamins are at fault, they abandon their intended regimens. In many cases, stomach upset results from a negative reaction to the substances used to fill out, bind, seal, or encapsulate the vitamin. Products with high concentrations of the chemical unpronounceables, e.g. polyvinylpyrridoline, are often at fault. Not even nutrient binders and fillers escape indictment. Lactose, a milk sugar indigestible to many adults, is a frequent culprit. Sucrose (table sugar), sorbitol, vegetable coloring, mannitol, agar, lecithin, brewers yeast, alfalfa, bran, and beeswax are common binders, fillers, and encapsulators that may cause distress in susceptible individuals. New laws require that supplement products list inactive as well as active ingredients in their formulation. Paying close attention to all labeling information—not only vitamin and mineral content—is important. By changing brands—if necessary—and by taking your supplements with or immediately after meals, you minimize the risk of upset and help ensure proper absorption—particularly of vitamins A, D, and E, which must dissolve in fat before crossing the intestinal wall.

DELIVERY FORMS

Because vitamins are comparatively fragile substances subject to deterioration on exposure to heat, light, and air, they are compounded and packaged in a fashion intended to maintain potency for the longest periods of time. Your choice of delivery form should be decided by a combination of factors—including ease of consumption, digestive tolerance, and economic considerations.

- *Tablets* are generally the most stable. Because of the protective effect provided by their binders and fillers, single-vitamin and multivitamin supplements, containing both water- and fat-soluble vitamins, are most frequently compounded in this form.

- *Capsules* enclosing the fat-soluble vitamins avoid the potentially unpleasant taste of fish or vegetable oils in which A, D, and E are often dissolved. Because they completely surround their nutritionally active ingredients, capsules are less apt to contain preservatives but are more likely to be dyed[3] than their tablet counterparts. They are generally more expensive.

- *Timed-release* tablets or capsules are intended to deliver their vitamins in small but continuous quantities over a 6-to-8-hour period. Because water-soluble C and members of the B complex achieve maximum concentrations in the blood within 2 hours and then diminish rapidly, it is argued that a sustained-release system can provide you with the advantage of relatively steady blood quantities of the various vitamins throughout the day. Because of differences in diges-

---

3. Powdered vitamins in capsule form generally do not have an unpleasant taste. By emptying the capsule and combining its dry content with foods you avoid unwanted dyes and potential problems with swallowing.

tive and absorptive processes from individual to individual, too many products release their vitamin content prematurely or not at all—particularly those relying on digestive enzymes or acidity for their action. Those triggered by water absorption from the gut appear reliable, but unless the variety of time release is indicated on a supplement label you cannot be certain that you will receive and absorb all the vitamins that are your due.

● *Liquid* forms work well for children and adults who have difficulty in downing tablets or capsules. They have the added advantage of flexibility—since you can control your level of supplementation by the volume you drink at any given time. They provide an attractive supplement alternative—so long as they don't contain alcohol as a solvent.

● *Drops* are primarily intended for infants but can be used to good effect by adults who have trouble swallowing or wish more latitude in adjusting their vitamin intake than allowed by pre-measured tablets or capsules.

● *Crystals* of calcium, potassium, or sodium ascorbate offer the purest, least expensive means of getting your vitamin C. They have a pleasant "fruity" taste when dissolved in a glass of water or orange juice. Since you can adjust the quantity of crystals to whatever level of intake you choose, you are not limited to standard formulations of 100, 250, 500, or 1,000 mg. In addition, ascorbate crystals will not acidify the digestive tract—a factor that can eliminate the problem of flatulence or diarrhea experienced by some users of ascorbic acid.

QUALITY CONTROL AND POTENCY

The FDA monitors both the labeling practices and content validity of all vitamin products. Frequent, random, and unannounced checks are run on all supplements.

Because some deterioration is normal for stored products, all manufacturers are allowed to include a margin of additional potency for each vitamin at the time of formulation. Failure to maintain claimed concentration, quality of composition, or standards of labeling results in loss of marketing approval.

IRRELEVANT INGREDIENTS

Although it is difficult to convince a biochemist that those vitamins manufactured in a laboratory are chemically different from or inferior to those extracted from so-called natural sources, claimed superiority for "organic" products may have a basis in fact. All too often synthesized vitamins are surrounded by binders, fillers, and coatings that introduce extraneous—even toxic—substances into the human digestive tract. That a nationally popular and otherwise rational vitamin/mineral formulation should have its nutritionally active ingredients surrounded by the following irrelevant substances beggars the imagination:

Anhydrous citric acid, carnauba wax, edible white ink, ethylcellulose, FD & C [Food Dye & Colorant] Blue #2, FD & C Red #3, FD & C Yellow #6, hydroxypropyl methylcellulose, polysorbate 80, polyvinylpyrridoline, propylene glycol, refined sugar, silicon dioxide, titanium dioxide, and vanillin.

Because their users demand it, most manufacturers of "natural" vitamin products are careful to avoid non-nutritive waxes, dyes, polishes, and other such chemical miscreants in their formulations. They *do* more often tend to exploit the belief that "more must be better" by including nutritionally irrelevant substances in their supplements. Such exotica as amino acids (e.g. lysine, betaine, glutamic acid, etc.), RNA, enzymes, essential fatty acids and the like[4] have no rational place in a vitamin/mineral product

---

4. Intrinsic factor—needed for the absorption of vitamin B_{12}—is an exception to this general rule.

—particularly in those trace concentrations in which they are usually included. They add substantially to your cost without benefiting your health.

PRE-PLANNING YOUR PURCHASE OF A VITAMIN SUPPLEMENT

- Before undertaking any program of vitamin supplementation you are wise to consult a knowledgeable and sympathetic physician.[5] Seek his advice and consider any reservations he may have based on his knowledge of your unique medical history.

- Do not under any circumstances embark on a supplementation regimen with the intent and purpose of "curing" any illness or disorder, no matter how trivial. Your only legitimate use of vitamins is as a food supplement intended to enrich your diet and subsequently your health. Nothing could be more foolhardy than to attempt your own treatment of a disorder with increased dosages of vitamins once symptoms of illness have appeared. Your physician is superbly trained to treat the bodily crises caused by disease. Don't second-guess or delay seeing him when ill. He needs to know about your use of vitamins since supplementation may affect the action of drugs he prescribes or alter the results of laboratory tests he may perform. (See Appendix A.)

- Plan your regimen with a clear understanding of your goals. *Do you simply intend to meet appropriate RDA requirements with a single supplement, allowing your diet to provide an additional margin of safety?* If so, you are probably wiser to consult the more flexible and more precise table of values provided by

---

5. There is no law against asking relevant questions of a physician. If his answers betray little knowledge of nutrition and the importance of vitamins, he is of value to you only as a curative or carative rather than a preventive practitioner. See Appendix A.

the Food and Nutrition Board (RDAs), than the cruder instrument promulgated by the FDA (U.S. RDAs). *Do you intend to follow a program ensuring higher levels of tissue concentration than provided by traditional RDAs?* If so, carefully consider the regimens included in Chapter 5, or other reputable programs from respected sources.

● Be sure to evaluate your potential vitamin needs in terms of your age, sex, body build, height, weight, personal history, and lifestyle.

● Review your diet with care. Can you eliminate all or a portion of the highly refined or processed foods? Sugar? Bleached flour? Processed oils? Caffeine? Cola drinks? If you consume foods particularly rich in various vitamins, e.g. brewers yeast, wheat germ, beef liver, adjust your supplementation accordingly.

After careful consideration of the foregoing, be sure to use Appendix D to plan your supplementation—before arriving at the vitamin counter.

CAVEATS AND CAUTIONS

● Remember that nutritional experts of all persuasions agree that vitamins function interdependently, are no more efficient than their least effective or concentrated member, and exert their positive effects slowly over a period of months, years, and decades. In principle, supplementation should be *comprehensive, consistent, and continuous.* Exaggerated intake of any one vitamin is futile. Overkill with fat-soluble vitamins may lead to poisoning. Excesses of water-soluble vitamins are rapidly excreted, but in the extreme may actually interfere with rather than support the functioning of other vitamins.

● Plan to take a basic supplement containing *all* the vitamins, reserving single or incomplete multiples to compensate for any deficiency in the multivitamin of your choice.

- Once you have selected a fundamental regimen, turn to the product charts in Appendix D. The formulations of more than 700 of the most common multivitamin, multivitamin/multimineral, and single-vitamin products are listed alphabetically by brand name. Find 3 to 4 multivitamin products that most nearly meet your needs. Use the single-ingredient charts to select any additional vitamin concentrations necessary to fulfill your proposed regimen. Consider whether tablets, capsules, liquids, or drops have any bearing on your choice.

- Be careful not to confuse micrograms (mcg or μg) with milligrams (mg) or grams (g).

- Take this book with its copy of your proposed regimen—along with the names of the alternative products you have selected—to your pharmacy, health food store, or vitamin outlet. Find those brands you have pre-selected. Check the labels with care (formulations do change) and compare their values in terms of cost. Vitamin supplementation can be expensive, particularly for the careless consumer. Higher prices are typical of nationally advertised brand-name products. Choose such supplements if you feel more comfortable with a well-known trade name behind you, but remember that unfamiliar or generically labeled products can provide you with equivalent quality and value for your dollar.[6]

- If necessary, and fortified with an appropriate grain of salt, enlist the aid of a salesperson or pharmacist. Don't be impressed by claims for natural or organic products—but don't necessarily reject them either. Your prior preparation should stay any impulse to buy that higher-priced formulation with its mystery ingredients. You are ready for the vitamin marketplace.

---

6. Many mail order houses offer excellent vitamin values and convenience in ordering.

VITAMINS & YOU
1980s Update

Appendix A

Vitamins & Your Physician

The elimination of death by infection is a 20th-century medical miracle that has profoundly altered national disease patterns. Heart and circulatory disorders, the many varieties of cancer, and complications arising from diabetes now constitute the primary causes of mortality in our modern industrial society. Although 30 years have passed since these chronic, degenerative, and non-infectious illnesses have become our primary killers, only marginal progress has been made toward their prevention and elimination—despite billions of man-hours and dollars spent on the development of more elaborate medical hardware, powerful drugs, and sophisticated scalpels. There has been progress to be sure. Breakthroughs in organ transplantation, heart valve replacement, microsurgery, and the use of laser beams were medical high points of the last decade; however, many argue that surgery has gone "just about as far as it can go," with future development more a matter of refinement than revolution. The many new classes of medication—including mood-altering drugs, diuretics, amphetamines, and painkillers—are of far less certain ben-

181

efit than their antibiotic and serum predecessors, as unintended dependence on prescription medications and severe drug side effects emerge as a major health-care problem. Overuse of surgery and prescription medications has spawned a whole new disease category—the *iatrogenic,* or physician-caused illness. It killed an estimated 180,000 Americans in 1980 and injured many more.

Criticism of the "all-eggs-in-two-baskets" approach to current medical research became highly vocal in the 1970s. After years of automatic funding, Congress called the scientific establishment to fiscal account, demanding that other lines of inquiry—including the nutritional—be vigorously pursued. At the individual level, growing numbers of physicians, frustrated by the limitations of prescription pad and scalpel, have begun to add non-surgical, non-drug therapies to their practice. Respected medical techniques from foreign medicine, e.g. acupuncture, and such innovative methodologies as biofeedback are gaining wide physician interest and acceptance. To the medical futurist this quest for therapeutic alternatives is the wave of the 80s: one that promises *holistic* practice drawing on a wide range of disciplines for preventing and curing disease, including diet, yoga, vitamin therapy, immune system manipulation—as well as drugs and surgery.

Although physician interest in nutrition—particularly vitamin nutrition—is considerable, it is difficult to apply in practice because the standard American medical school curriculum virtually ignores the subject. Postgraduate attempts to gain nutritional insight are often frustrating because information is currently fragmentary, often contradictory, or simply nonexistent. However, necessary involvement with epidemic obesity, the low-cholesterol diet recommended for cardiac patients, and the need to manage diabetic nutrition is making our physicians potent spokesmen for the development of a rigorous nutritional science.

Whether your medical doctor belongs to the growing category of nutritionally responsive physicians is often a matter of the purest chance. Indeed, his or her reaction to your personal concern about nutrition—particularly ade-

quate or optimum vitamin nutrition—may prove a useful
index of his or her value to you as a preventive (as well
as a curative or carative) health-care advisor. Being told
to "Get all the vitamins you need with your knife and
fork" should not satisfy your legitimate demand to pursue
all reasonable means for preventing disease before it starts.
Diagnostic tools now exist that can satisfy your physician's requirements for a rigorous approach to evaluating
vitamin needs. An alert practitioner will be ready to listen
and work with you toward the goal of optimal health.

VITAMIN LAB TESTS AND YOUR M.D.

In this age of highly technological medicine, most
physicians feel uncomfortable about making recommendations to patients that are not in some way based on data
from specific laboratory tests. Although an average of 1
such medical procedure in 4 yields inaccurate or misleading results due to human or technical error, physicians
continue to rely on such techniques because they *do* often
provide valuable information, appear "scientific," and
offer a measure of legal protection against charges of mal-
practice (when therapy has been predicated on the results
of such tests).

Unfortunately—despite highly refined procedures for
measuring body levels of sugars, fats, and proteins; numerous drugs; and various nutritional byproducts—laboratory methods for determining an individual's vitamin
status have remained comparatively primitive, time consuming, and unreliable. The absence of such desirable
diagnostic tools has made it traditionally difficult, if not
impossible, for physicians to obtain objective data about
their patients' specific vitamin health and requirements
and does much to explain professional hesitancy about the
use of supplements. Such reluctance may become obsolete
as new analytic techniques—now available to the medical
profession—make possible more precise and reliable vitamin evaluations.

Although it would be diagnostically *ideal* to measure vitamin quantities inside the cells and tissues where the biochemical business of life is transacted, knowledge of blood levels for these nutrients can potentially tell your physician a great deal about your vitamin status. A new test, developed by research chemists at the New Jersey Medical School, does just that by measuring blood concentrations of the nine recognized water-soluble and two of the fat-soluble vitamins (D and K escape detection). The test requires your physician to draw a blood sample, which must be forwarded to—

College of Medicine and Dentistry of New Jersey
New Jersey Medical School
Vitamin Assay Center
88 Ross Street
East Orange, New Jersey
07018

Results are normally returned within a week along with a consultative interpretation of the findings. The cost is $10 for single vitamin determinations, e.g. folic acid level, or $75 for the complete battery.

Because the test is so new, your physician may be unfamiliar with it. He or she can obtain more information about the procedure by writing directly to the Assay Center or by phoning (201) 456–6565. As with all laboratory procedures, awareness of the test's limitations and potential for misinterpretation is important. For example, your use of supplements prior to drawing of the blood will undoubtably mask evidence of deficiency. Similarly, during periods of nutritional deprivation the results may appear unjustifiably positive. Blood levels may register as normal or even elevated because cells and tissues may be breaking down and releasing their vitamins for circulatory system transport and use by other vital tissues and organs. Careful attention to such factors is critical if your physician is to make an accurate determination of your vitamin status using this potentially invaluable diagnostic tool.

Another new procedure for determining vitamin concentrations is now available to your medical doctor or dentist. Although the test measures only ascorbic acid levels, it is of importance because of growing recognition of vitamin C's multifaceted role in the maintenance of good health. The procedure simply requires that a drop of test solution be deposited on the tongue. The time it takes to lose its characteristic blue color reveals relative tissue concentrations of the vitamin, e.g. an elapsed time of 20 seconds or less indicates that tissue is well supplied with C; 20 to 25 seconds suggests the presence of only marginal ascorbic acid levels; and 25 or more seconds reflects a pronounced deficiency state. The advantages of this technique, known as the Lingual Ascorbic Acid Test (LAAT), are that it measures actual tissue concentrations for the vitamin (rather than blood, urine, or saliva levels); is inexpensive; and can be performed by any medical professional—physician, dentist, lab technician, or nurse—in less than 1 minute. The test, originally developed by research physicians at the University of Alabama Medical Center, is obtainable in kit form, along with a complete bibliography, from—

Medical Diagnostics Services, Inc.
P.O. Box 1441
Brandon, Florida
33511

Although both the blood assay and the Lingual Ascorbic Acid Test require administration by trained technicians, there are at least 2 procedures that you can use at home for estimating your individual nutrient status. One is a simple test-stick that rapidly and accurately reveals vitamin C concentrations in body fluids. It involves a specially coated, throwaway plastic strip that turns color —ranging from pale yellow to dark blue—on exposure to various concentrations of vitamin C in a drop of urine. This inexpensive dip-and-read test is marketed under the brand name C-Stix and is available either directly from your pharmacist in bottles of 50 strips or from—

Specialty Systems Department
Ames Company
(Division of Miles Laboratories, Inc.)
Elkart, Indiana
46514

Regular use of C-Stix can accurately monitor vitamin C requirements so that you can adjust supplementation to meet your exact needs at any given time. A less precise but useful personal test is a simple visual examination of urine color. A vibrant, almost metallic yellow indicates that you are excreting large surplus quantities of vitamin C and that you can cut back your supplementation until only a trace of this characteristic color is regularly visible. Similarly, an intense green suggests excretion of abundant quantities of B-complex vitamins. Reducing your supplementation so that only a slight hint of this typical green is evident will help assure optimum vitamin nutrition without waste.

Although these methods for personal vitamin assessment are less than perfect, they can be of considerable use to both you and your physician.

MINERALS AND YOUR M.D.

Many individuals—medical professionals as well as laymen—tend to think of vitamins and minerals as nutritionally synonymous. The assumption is understandable. Both nutrient groups are essential for life in minute quantities, share many similar co-enzyme functions that regulate body chemistry, produce severe—even lethal—disease if inadequately supplied, and must be continuously fed to the body from outside sources (since neither can be manufactured by human metabolic machinery). However, there are also very major differences between vitamins and minerals that must be understood to avoid potential nutritional injury. Vitamins are extremely fragile organic substances that can only be synthesized by living cells—the plant or animal cells of the foods we eat[1] or the microbes that live in our digestive tract. All are necessary to life. All can be easily destroyed by harsh chemical and physical handling—whether through food processing, cooking, or intestinal upset. All are biochemically amiable, with water-soluble varieties producing few, if any, side effects in virtually any amounts and fat-soluble varieties causing no more than mild and reversible toxicity in only wildly exaggerated quantities.

Minerals—in striking contrast— are hardy elements that do not break down with rough usage. Not only are they supplied by the foods we eat but also by the water we drink. Of the more than 100 minerals (or elements) known to science, fewer than 25 are essential to human metabolism. Many of the remaining 75-plus are highly poisonous and potentially dangerous. A fine balance must be struck among those necessary to life processes or serious biochemical injury may result. Among those minerals essential to humans in relatively large amounts are calcium (Ca), magnesium (Mg), phosphorus (P), sodium (Na), potassium (K), iron (Fe), and copper (Cu). Also critical—but in much smaller concentrations—are the trace minerals: zinc (Zn), manganese (Mn), molybdenum (Mo), chromium (Cr), selenium (Se), lithium (Li), Nickel (Ni), vanadium (V), and cobalt (Co). Among those non-essential and frequently toxic elements that may easily build up in the tissues of 20th-century Americans are mercury (Hg), aluminum (Al), cadmium (Cd), arsenic (As), and palladium (Pd).

Although there is increasing evidence that mineral inadequacy or imbalance is a cause for many medical problems—iron deficiency among menstruating women probably being the most widely known—it is simply not reasonable *to estimate* your mineral status and needs without very specific laboratory tests. While it is possible to predict your dietary intake of other essential elements, unless you know the mineral content of the water you

---

1. They may ultimately find their way to the byproducts of such cells, e.g. milk, fat, starches, or sugars.

drink it is virtually impossible to assess the quantities you regularly ingest or excrete, i.e. those that may be oversupplied, undersupplied, or in improper balance. Without precise testing you are wise to limit your supplementary intake of all minerals—so often included with desired vitamins in multiple products—to no more than U.S. RDA quantities.

If you do suspect that mineral imbalance is a personal problem, there are reliable steps that *you and your physician* together can take to accurately determine your nutrient status. Although blood and urine tests will provide considerable information, the most comprehensive and useful mineral data come from hair analyses *provided by professional and licensed laboratories.* Unfortunately, too many part-time chemists have set up home laboratories and advertise hair analysis for a fee. The usual practice is for a consumer to mail in a curly lock and a substantial check along with a self-addressed and stamped envelope. All too often there are no clear instructions about how to cut the sample, nor considerations of important data such as age, height, sex, weight, or factors of personal habit such as use of hair coloring, specific shampoos, bleaches, or dyes. Results returned to the unsuspecting may or may not be chemically accurate or relevant and can lead to serious problems if any attempt is made to correct "mineral imbalance" without professional assistance.

Because properly gathered and interpreted data can reveal a great deal about your mineral health, it is wise to seek that information in conjunction with your physician. Indeed, the most reputable laboratories will only accept hair samples submitted by an M.D. Their detailed analyses of your exact concentrations of the 7 major minerals, 9 trace minerals, and half-dozen or so commonly toxic elements is returned to your physician with specific interpretation, suggested means for increasing deficient nutrient concentrations through diet or supplementation, methods for correcting imbalances between elements (e.g. calcium and magnesium, sodium and potassium), and possible means for eliminating excessive quantities of toxic elements. In this way—and this way only—can you and your physician be reasonably certain of an accurate understanding of your mineral health.

Because hair analysis is viewed with justifiable suspicion by many medical professionals, your physician may not know of reputable laboratories. Among those that will undoubtably meet his or her critical standards are

MineraLab, Inc.
3501 Breakwater Avenue
Hayward, California
94545

MineraLab, Inc.
409 Massachusetts Avenue
Acton, Massachusetts
01720

DRUGS AND YOUR VITAMIN STATUS

Given modern medicine's propensity for the prescription pad, it is not surprising that most adult Americans take physician-ordered medications every day. Because the vast majority of drugs in common use are synthetic in origin, most are chemically alien to human metabolism and must be detoxified by vitamin C– and B-complex–dependent enzyme systems in the liver. Many are injurious to sensitive mucous linings of the digestive tract—interfering with the proper absorption of vital nutrients, e.g. vitamins and minerals, from the gut, or destroying the important intestinal microbes that normally manufacture essential vitamins. The result of regularly consuming medication can, therefore, become a significantly increased personal need for specific vitamins—particularly the water-soluble varieties.

Although the complex relationship among drugs, nutritional status, and vitamins is a relatively unexplored field, it is imperative that you and your physician realize that daily medication can impair your nutritional health and is capable of producing serious vitamin deficiencies. Because drug-induced *mal*nutrition tends to develop slowly and insidiously, it is not always easy to recognize. Be on the alert for—

● oral contraceptives, which drain the body's supplies of vitamins B_6, folic acid, C, and E.

- mineral oil and other laxatives, which reduce the absorption of fat-soluble vitamins and many minerals.

- antibiotics, particularly neomycin, which decrease the absorption of vitamins A, K, folic acid, and B_{12}, sodium, calcium, potassium, iron, nitrogen, various sugars, and essential fats.

- cholesterol-lowering drugs, which reduce body levels of vitamins A, K, D, and B_{12}, iron, and glucose.

- analgesics, which limit absorption of folic acid, fats, and vitamin B_{12}.

- diuretics and antacids, which deplete supplies of water-soluble vitamins and minerals.

- tetracycline antibiotics, which increase your need for C and destroy important intestinal microbes.

As a general rule: Don't accept any prescription for long-term medication without closely questioning your physician about its potential for damaging your nutritional well-being and the wisdom of taking supplementary vitamins and minerals to compensate for the kinds of damages that potentially accompany your drug therapy.

SOURCES FOR NUTRITIONALLY ORIENTED MEDICAL PROFESSIONALS

Although increasing numbers of physicians, dentists, and psychiatrists are actively incorporating nutritional therapies—particularly programs of vitamin and mineral supplementation—into their medical practices, it is not always easy to find qualified practitioners. The following organizations publish national directories of nutritionally oriented health-care professionals that are available to you on written request:

American Academy of Medical
Preventics
2811 L Street
Suite 205
Sacramento, California
95816

Directory of Nutrition-Minded
Drs. (U.S. and Canada, $1.00)
c/o Alacer Corporation
Buena Park, California
90622

Huxley Institute for Biosocial
Research
1114 First Avenue
New York, New York
10021

International Academy of
Preventive Medicine
10409 Town and Country Way
Houston, Texas
77024

International Academy of
Metabology
P.O. Box 15157
Las Cruces, New Mexico
88001

International College of Applied
Nutrition
Box 386
La Habra, California
90631

International Foundation for
Preventive Medicine
6932-B Little River Turnpike
Annandale, Virginia
22003

Orthomolecular Medical Society
2698 Pacific Avenue
San Francisco, California
94115

Appendix B

Breakthroughs: The Therapeutic Use of Vitamins in the 80s

"Can vitamins cure disease?" is one of the most often asked and least satisfactorily answered medical questions of the age. In the absence of hard and fast evidence, there can be no certainty about the effectiveness of vitamin therapies. Any verdict—whether rendered by government agency, physician, nutritionist, research scientist, or vitamin enthusiast—is today a matter of conjecture rather than absolute medical truth. Fortunately, the coming decade promises to resolve much of the contention, controversy, and confusion about the therapeutic uses of vitamins while dispelling much of the myth, mystique, and illusion currently surrounding supplementation. The reasons are many—

THE RESEARCH MORATORIUM

Between 1920 and 1950 enthusiasm for nutritional studies among scientists was at fever pitch. Successful identification, isolation, or synthesis of a particular vitamin often generated a Nobel Prize or similar honor for the biochemist. Recognition that minimal concentrations of these nutrients are essential to all life led to speculation that increased intake would confer important health benefits on the human body. Optimistic reports in the scientific literature brought a lavish expenditure of research time and money. Investigators—intent on discovering another group of wonder drugs equivalent to antibiotics and sulfanilamides—were, however, thwarted in their efforts to bend supplementary vitamins into therapeutic tools capable of curing such then dread diseases as polio. The best evidence—generated through undeniably careful research —*seemed* irrefutable:

> By maintaining adequate supplies of dietary vitamins, all of the depletion disorders, i.e. scurvy, rickets, pellagra, etc., can be avoided. Increasing intake beyond the levels adequate to escape such diseases has little discernible effect on any other disease.

This summary research view has prevailed for more than 30 years in the traditional medical and nutritional thinking, training, and textbooks of physicians, dietitians, and health care officials.

That the time, labor, and money spent on postwar vitamin studies seemed wasted to the scientific establishment is understandable and does much to explain reluctance to fund further research. Indeed, the Old Boy method for allocating federal grant monies on the unilateral recommendation of a single, senior research scientist —many of whom had been disappointed by early vitamin studies—put an effective lid on American nutritional research for more than 3 decades. Replacement of that autocratic system in the mid 1970s through the direct intervention of Congress reopened government coffers to any and all defensible research questions. Investigators—now less shackled by funding bias—could resume nutritional inquiries, armed with far finer biochemical tools than their predecessors, stimulated by the findings of foreign scientists, and aware that the unproductive outcome of previous research may have resulted from using too little of a given vitamin for too short a time and for inappropriate purposes.

Although 5 years is a very brief period for laboratory research, preliminary findings indicate that long-cherished beliefs held by all combatants on the vitamin battlefront will undergo considerable modification. The eminent physician who recently articulated the traditional view that he knew "no legitimate use for vitamins other than the prevention or cure of deficiency diseases such as scurvy" will find his horizons measurably widened. Similarly, the ardent vitamin advocate will abandon many of the biochemically unsound—potentially injurious—enthusiasms for vitamin treatments and therapies that have attracted Americans as kids to the cookie jar. We are undeniably moving from an era of vitamin rhetoric to one of solid vitamin research.

THERAPEUTIC BREAKTHROUGHS IN THE 80s

On the basis of evidence in hand, it is fascinating to speculate—in Jules Verne fashion—about some of the possible vitamin breakthroughs that may occur in the coming decade. Some will predictably be confirmed, some denied.

Heart and Circulatory Disorders

Heart disease became a "nutritional disorder" in the 1960s when studies revealed a close correlation between blood levels of cholesterol and the occurrence of coronaries, strokes, and other cardiovascular "accidents." Population studies apparently confirmed the link since in countries where diets are cholesterol rich—the United States and Finland—the incidence of heart disease is epidemic, while nations enjoying a low-cholesterol menu—Japan—suffer a moderate to rare occurrence of such disorders.

Although scientists know that coincidence does not prove cause and effect, physicians and the American public have proclaimed a war on dietary cholesterol as the principal villain in heart and circulatory disease.

During the 1970s the nutritionally responsive and concerned citizen dutifully reduced his consumption of cholesterol-laden animal fats, replacing them with polyunsaturated vegetable shortening and oils. The anticipated decline in blood levels of cholesterol and control of heart disease largely failed to materialize for reasons that seem to baffle the physician and medical establishment. Ignorance of basic nutrition is at fault, and no more compelling case can be made for the subject's intensive study in medical school than this 15-year folly.

Although solid deposits of cholesterol undoubtedly reduce the diameter of blood vessels, impair circulation, elevate blood pressure, and help cause heart attack and stroke, elimination of the molecule from the diet does not eliminate it from the body. Cholesterol in food is chemically dismembered by our digestive processes before it passes into the circulatory system. The liver uses these molecular fragments as grist to its biochemical mill, often converting these and other molecular fragments into many different kinds of compound—including cholesterol —depending on its immediate needs and demands. If dietary supplies are lacking, the liver will transform varying quantities of carbohydrates or unsaturated oils into the cholesterol the body requires for normal biological functioning. Because the liver is in biochemical command, it is hardly surprising that the elimination of dietary cholesterol has little impact on blood levels of the compound.

Convincing but often overlooked evidence has for years linked the quantities of cholesterol in the blood to hereditary factors, body weight, age, sex, exercise, and personal habits such as smoking and drinking. Similar evidence suggests that a critical ratio between dietary calories and the vitamins needed for their metabolic processing is essential to keep blood cholesterol at a personal minimum. Diets rich in fat of any kind require quantities of vitamin C to control cholesterol and triglyceride formation, while those rich in polyunsaturates demand the addition of vitamin E. The proper metabolism of protein relies on appropriate supplies of the B vitamins—particularly B_2 and B_6—while carbohydrate utilization is heavily dependent on supplies of vitamin B_1 and pantothenic acid.

Recent and intriguing research indicates that the formation of cholesterol deposits on blood-vessel walls is as much linked to the health of the wall as it is to the quantities of cholesterol in the blood that passes through it. Cross-sectional studies confirm the basic physical fact that the smoother a conduit's surface, the less frictional resistance it offers to the fluids it carries. In the case of arteries and capillaries, cholesterol deposits (called plaques) occur with far greater frequency on rough or uneven vessel linings that offer increased frictional resistance to blood flow. Because smoothness of the arterial wall depends on the presence of healthy *ground substance*—a kind of biochemical glue that coats blood vessels and holds them together—its chemistry has been intensively investigated. Studies reveal that lubricating ability is directly correlated with available quantities of vitamin C and that continuous supplies of the nutrient are essential. However, ground substance yields biochemical precedence to the adrenal glands, which demand enormous quantities of C for the manufacture of "stress" hormones. The hypertensive or chronically ill live in a more-or-less permanent state of stress, which burdens the adrenal glands and continuously pressures the arterial ground substance to release its vitamin C. Prolonged withdrawal of C for emergency hormone synthesis evidently results in a local deficiency that can ultimately disrupt the vessel lining, making it susceptible to plaque formation.

This fundamental biochemical mechanism suggests an impressive correlation among stress, high blood pressure, cholesterol levels, plaque formation, and sub-clinical vitamin C deficiency in arterial walls. Further studies are needed, but what is now known offers considerable hope for a major breakthrough in the prevention and cure of heart and circulatory disorders in the 1980s.

Cancer

Barely a week passes without the media's reporting that another common chemical in the environment causes cancer in laboratory animals. Of the more than 6,000 substances so far tested, more than 2,000 demonstrate carcinogenic, or cancer-causing, capacities. Although rodents—the test animals—are an imperfect proxy for man, we are close biochemical relatives, and it is scientifically reasonable to assume that a significant number of substances are carcinogenic for both of us.

Public awareness that cancer-causing substances permeate our environment is practically universal. That health-care officials offer little advice about how to avoid such substances—other than to stop smoking and to eat plenty of roughage—leaves many Americans with a sense that the development of cancer is a kind of blind lottery over which they have little control.

Although continuing contact with carcinogens is probably inevitable, only 1 in 5 ever develops the disease. That 80 percent escape malignancy is fascinating as it suggests the body is ordinarily capable of neutralizing the ubiquitous cancer-causing chemicals it encounters daily, and that an exceptional breakdown in the defense system may account for the 20 percent incidence of the disease. Because 25 years may elapse between exposure to a cancer-causing agent and symptoms of malignancy, proof of a definite cause and effect between a suspected carcinogen and cancer is difficult; however, biochemical inquiry into possible means by which the body might protect itself from cancer-causing agents has been in progress for 40 years. Evidence now exists that there are many carcinogen-resisting mechanisms. All involve specific vitamins.

Although there are many varieties of cancer, about 90 percent of them develop along the mucous membranes lining the nose, mouth, throat, lungs, and digestive tract. The concentrated incidence of malignancy among these tissues is not surprising since they form the first and most concentrated point of contact for the exchange of materials between the external world and the body itself. These membranes have long been recognized as an effective barrier against microbes, rarely breaking down and allowing infection to enter the system. They are equally efficient chemical and physical filters that trap alien and toxic substances unless weakened by repeated assaults of the kind caused by smoking.

Because the health of mucous membranes is undeniably dependent on continuous supplies of vitamin A (retinol) and vitamin C (ascorbic acid), many investigators in the 1980s—including the head of the National Cancer Institute (NCI)—identify these two compounds and their chemical relatives as the currently most promising agents for the prevention and possible cure of cancers.

Evidently, the anti-cancer properties of retinol and ascorbic acid extend beyond their involvement in maintaining the health of mucous linings. Both can prevent the transformation of potential carcinogens into actual cancer-causing compounds. For example, substances called nitrites have long been added to bacon, luncheon meat, ham, and sausage—imparting characteristic redness and providing critical protection against bacterial spoilage. Unfortunately, nitrites are chemically converted into highly carcinogenic *nitrosamines* on contact with the heat of cooking. In the presence of vitamin C this transformation does not occur, and the U.S. Department of Agriculture has recently ordered the addition of ascorbic acid—or one of its chemical relatives—to any meat that continues to be cured with nitrite. Nature has long provided similar protection to fruits and vegetables, which contain large quantities of substances called nitrates. These compounds would also become nitrosamines were it not for the natural vitamin C content of such produce. Because warehouse storage results in considerable loss of vitamin C, legislation requiring the addition of C to supermarket fruits and vegetables may soon be necessary.

Although it is vitamins A and C that will attract the greatest cancer research attention in the 80s, other vitamins—notably the B complex and E—have stirred considerable interest. Attention focuses on the liver as the body's biochemical clearinghouse. Among its thousands of functions is its critical role in ridding the system of poisonous waste products and any alien chemicals—including carcinogens—that may get into the bloodstream. Detoxification is dependent on chemical reactions that principally rely on B-complex vitamins working together as a team. Other neutralizing activities involve vitamin E and ascorbic acid, with the latter playing an additional and critical role in the functioning of the white blood cells that can and do attack malignant tissue once it forms.

All vitamins will play a major role in cancer research during the coming decade. Their hypothetical potential for the prevention and cure of this disease is enormous. Their actual effectiveness remains to be proved.

Diabetes

Biochemical difficulty in metabolizing sugar and other carbohydrates is a common problem among Americans. Although abnormalities arise from a number of different causes, most forms are described by the umbrella term *diabetes.* None is more severe than that suffered by the young, who apparently inherit a defective gene for the production of insulin, the pancreatic hormone needed to chemically process dietary sugars. Treatment requires daily, lifelong injections of the hormone. More prevalent is the "late-onset" form, typical of 80 percent of American diabetics. It is a disorder whose symptoms usually surface in middle age and evidently result—not necessarily from a lack of insulin production—but from the loss of ability to absorb sufficient quantities of the hormone into vital cells and tissues. Control over the late-onset disorder can usually be achieved by careful attention to diet, weight control, exercise, and in many cases the daily intake of oral insulin.

Because medical management of the various forms of the disease is normally uncomplicated and allows the diabetic a nearly normal life, many physicians and patients tend to minimize the problems it poses. However, it is clear that the older diabetic—following years of evidently successful treatment—is unusually susceptible to heart and circulatory diseases, cancer, nervous system disorders, infection, kidney failure, cataracts, and blindness. Therapy that keeps a patient symptom-free and perfectly functional apparently does not prevent subtle injury to various organs because of a sub-clinical and progressive erosion in the health of the tiny capillaries that link arteries with veins in all tissue.

Because an average of 18 years elapses between the onset of diabetic symptoms and evidence of severe secondary illness, tissue damage is often profound and irreversible before detection. These delayed complications now make diabetes the third most lethal disease, after circulatory disorders and cancer.

A concerted research effort is predictably underway to identify the causes of sub-clinical capillary deterioration during the long first stage of diabetes. Because of its critical role in maintaining the health of blood vessel linings, vitamin C—at levels of tissue saturation in conjunction with its close biochemical relatives, the bioflavonoids —holds considerable promise for deferring or preventing the ultimate diabetic injury and death. It is already clear that supplementary quantities of C make insulin more effective—possibly by promoting its passage across cell membranes—and can lower the quantities of hormone needed to regulate carbohydrate metabolism.

Arthritis

Thirty-two million Americans currently suffer from one or another of the bone and joint diseases generally known as arthritis. Of these 16 million are afflicted by *osteoarthritis*—a degenerative condition typical of aging. It is a "wear and tear" disorder characterized by deterioration of the cartilage, which pads bone ends and makes possible the free movement of joints. As cushioning tissues lose their resilience, movement becomes increasingly painful and debilitating.

Because it produces little inflammation and swelling, osteoarthritis is considerably less severe than the *rheumatoid* forms that currently cripple 6.5 million of us.[1] Symptoms of the latter normally strike before 50 years of age, affect nearly three times as many women as men, and can produce the greatest injury—not only to joint tissue, but to all of the supportive ligaments, tendons, cartilage, and membranes that hold the body together. It characteristically causes swelling and intense inflammation of joint tissues without apparent cause—as the full force of the body's immune system inexplicably turns against the very tissue it normally protects. Repeated bouts of inflammation tend to grow progressively more severe and ultimately leave susceptible joints and other tissue permanently swollen and inoperable.

Like heart and circulatory disorders, cancer, and diabetes, the various forms of arthritis are diseases of Western civilization. Their incidence among people *of the same age group* in industrialized nations often exceeds that in underdeveloped countries by a factor of 5. Yet research science has failed to pinpoint the factors in our lifestyle or environment that stimulate this startling prevalence of degenerative disease. Virtually powerless to prevent the various forms of arthritis, a contemporary physician is only partially equipped to deal with overt symptoms once they appear. All recognized therapies involve the daily use of drugs (aspirin, Indocin, Motrin, steroids, etc.) that produce varying degrees of side effect ranging from the moderate to the severe. All suppress symptoms, none eliminates causes of disease.

Although dietary factors are logical targets for inquiry in the development of any chronic, debilitating disease, the 25-year moratorium on nutritional research has left much of American medicine at the mid-century mark. Fortunately, promising investigations in other countries are now being repeated and verified here. Many involve vitamin therapies for the prevention or amelioration of

---

1. Less common forms of arthritis, e.g. gout, osteoporosis, osteomalacia, lupus, afflict an estimated 9.5 million.

arthritic conditions. Most hopeful are procedures involving the use of pantothenic acid and niacin (niacinamide) to stimulate production of the body's own anti-inflammatory steroids and prostaglandins; pyridoxine and para aminobenzoic acid to promote joint flexibility; tocopherol and retinol to stimulate cartilage healing; synthetic calciferol to assist calcium absorption for proper bone formation; and vitamin C to suppress rheumatoid cells and accelerate the elimination of toxic metals that often aggravate arthritic conditions. Whether vitamin therapies for arthritic conditions will prove effective remains to be seen. That they are at last being given a day in court is reassuring.

Dentistry

It is a reasonable certainty that oral surgeons, periodontists, and other dental-care specialists will be the first medical professionals to adopt vitamin therapy as a routine preventative and therapeutic tool during the 1980s. The vitamin of choice will be C because of already persuasive evidence for its effectiveness in preventing tooth decay, retarding the formation of calculi, maintaining healthy gums, increasing the effectiveness of antibiotic medication, and helping stimulate repair of bone and connective tissue while accelerating the healing process following infection or surgery. Maximum benefit apparently occurs when tissue is saturated with the vitamin. Under-the-tongue (sublingual) tests for ascorbic acid levels are now available and help quickly determine the quantities of C you need to reach optimum tissue concentrations.

Drug Use and Abuse

Recent studies indicate that chronic drug use—licit or illicit—is one of the 10 primary causes of malnutrition among Americans. The biochemical reasons are simple. Most drugs—including alcohol—are alien to the body and must be chemically processed by the liver. This manipulation involves various groups of enzymes, all of which depend on vitamins for effective function. The regular intake of a drug places constant pressure on these enzyme systems and elevates the body's demand for dietary vitamins. For example, cholesterol-reducing drugs lower tissue levels of vitamins A, D, K, and B_{12}, while analgesics such as aspirin and aspirin substitutes increase the need for ascorbic acid. Some medications—e.g. mineral oils and other laxatives, antacids, and antibiotics—simply interfere with the absorption of fat-soluble vitamins (A, D, E, and K) from the small intestine. Others, e.g. diuretics, accelerate the normal flushing of water-soluble C and B-complex vitamins, often creating a temporary deficiency state. Recreational drugs such as cocaine attack specific tissues, e.g. the nasal membranes, which require additional quantities of vitamins A and C for their repair.[2]

More positive findings suggest that many drugs work more effectively at lower dosages if taken along with supplementary vitamins. This is true of aspirin, insulin, and many antibiotics simultaneously consumed with gram quantities of ascorbic acid. Evidently, the vitamin increases the activity of drug-metabolizing enzymes in the liver. This speeds breakdown of the medication and shortens the time it remains in the blood and tissue. In this fashion the vitamin reduces the chances for drug poisoning, other severe side effects, and adverse reactions.

More promising still is the current and experimental use of therapeutic vitamins to promote detoxification and tissue recovery among alcoholics, heroin addicts, and hyperactive children sensitive to refined sugars and common food additives.

While the coming decade promises us a rigorous nutritional science that will largely confirm or deny the benefits of therapeutic vitamin supplementation, waiting until the jury comes back is very much like anticipating

---

2. Injury to the mucous linings of throat and lung is typical of marijuana users. Tissue repair—if possible—is dependent upon increased concentrations of vitamins A, C, and the bioflavonoids.

the Surgeon General's Report on Smoking. We probably have 3 alternatives:

To maintain our dietary status quo, relying on a wide variety of foods to fulfill our personal nutritional needs,

or

To hedge all bets by supplementing our diets with RDA quantities of all the vitamins, while paying close attention to the quality of the foods we eat,

or

To attempt so-called optimum vitamin nutrition by maintaining tissue saturation with water-soluble B complex and C while achieving ample stores of fat-soluble A, D, and E without neglecting a well-balanced diet.

The choice is up to you. It is guaranteed by Congress and the 1975 "Freedom of Nutritional Choice Bill" that defines vitamins as foods, not drugs.

Appendix C

Vitamins & Your Health: The 50 Most Commonly Asked Questions

It has been my privilege in recent months to discuss vitamins, health, and nutrition on more than 300 radio and television programs in 26 cities across the United States and Canada. The following 50 questions were the most frequently asked by people from all walks of life.

AT WHAT TIME OF DAY SHOULD I TAKE MY SUPPLEMENTS?

You need vitamins to make the most efficient use of the foods you eat. Because they are such important food elements, it makes the best biological sense to take them along with meals. Breakfast is probably your best bet—before the peak activity and stress of your day. Whatever meal you choose, don't swallow supplements on an empty stomach if you can help it. By taking your vitamins along with food you minimize the risk of digestive upset while prolonging nutritional benefits, as food retards the passage of vitamins through your system and protects them from destruction by digestive juices.

HOW OFTEN SHOULD I TAKE MY VITAMINS?

To be nutritionally effective, any program of supplementation must be *comprehensive,* i.e. inclusive of all the vitamins—fat-soluble A, D, and E, and water-soluble C and members of the B complex; *concentrated,* i.e. taken in balanced quantities of sufficient strength to satisfy your body's optimum metabolic needs; and *continuous,* i.e. taken on a regular and consistent basis. Because your system will largely eliminate any surplus C and members of the B complex within 24 hours, you need your personal allowance of these vitamins on a daily basis. Because extra A, D, and/or E is stored by the liver for future use, it is possible to take these fat-soluble vitamins every second or third day in appropriate amounts. However, because optimum vitamin nutrition should become a positive factor in your daily lifestyle, it is probably wise to consume your personal allowance for all the vitamins every day.

NOTE: A supplement consumed casually—now and then—is apt to be a waste of time and money.

I'VE TRIED TAKING VITAMINS IN THE PAST BUT HAVE ALWAYS GIVEN UP BECAUSE THEY UPSET MY STOMACH, GIVE ME DIARRHEA, ARE HARD TO SWALLOW, AND TASTE TERRIBLE TO BOOT. CAN YOU HELP?

Taking your supplement along with other foods makes good nutritional sense and should help prevent digestive distress. If "vitamins at mealtimes" doesn't solve the problem, check the binders and fillers, which flesh out your supplement, and look for brands that deliver their active nutrients without such ingredients—e.g. lactose, one of the most frequent culprits.

Because most supplements provide their vitamin C in the form of ascorbic acid, a significant number of people suffer from diarrhea or apparent acid indigestion when taking the vitamin. If you are one of the sensitive who is upset by the mild acidification of ascorbic acid, look for brands that list non-acidifying *ascorbate* as their source for C.

NOTE: You no longer need to suffer from the agonizing taste of cod liver oil or the pungency of B-complex vitamins to get optimal nutrition. Gelatin capsules, coated tablets, and naturally flavored liquids or drops will deliver the vitamin nutrition you need without offending your taste buds.

WHERE SHOULD I STORE MY VITAMINS?

Because they are fragile substances that break down on contact with heat, light, and air, your supplements need the protection of a dry, dark, and cool environment. Most manufacturers help by enclosing their products in opaque containers that may or may not include an anti-moisture sachet or capsule (desiccant), absorbent cotton, a wax paper seal, and probable date of potency expiration (printed on the label). Because they are foods, it is logical to keep your supplements handy in the kitchen or dining room—but safely out of the reach of young children. The refrigerator or freezer, while dark and cool, is not a good storage choice because it often accumulates damaging moisture. Your spice rack may prove ideal because seasonings generally require the same conditions as vitamins to maintain freshness and potency.

I'VE STARTED TAKING VITAMINS AND MY URINE HAS TURNED A BRIGHT, ALMOST METALLIC YELLOW. I'M WORRIED.

Don't be. The color change can be startling but should cause no alarm. It indicates that you are excreting quantities of C that your body does not need. Cut back your daily intake until you observe no more than a trace of this highly characteristic color. Then you will know that you are achieving optimum concentrations of C without wasting your supplement. Similarly, a greenish urine indicates the flushing of surplus B-complex vitamins. Adjust your intake accordingly.

NOTE: There is no quicker way for instantly estimating *your* personal need for C or the B complex than these simple visual tests. (See Appendix A for a fuller discussion of vitamin test procedures.)

WHAT ARE RDAS? CAN I RELY ON THEM FOR GOOD HEALTH?

Recommended Dietary Allowances (RDAs) are periodic estimates made by a panel of "experts," i.e. the Food and Nutrition Board of the National Research Council, about your probable needs for various nutrients including protein, vitamins, and minerals. These quantities—held adequate to prevent such vitamin-deficiency disorders as scurvy, beri beri, rickets, and pellagra—are simplified and adapted by the Food and Drug Administration (FDA) as nutritional standards called U.S. RDAs. Labels on food products often bear a breakdown of their contents, listing the proportion of U.S. RDAs for protein, vitamins, and minerals delivered per serving or container.

For many years the Food and Nutrition Board enjoyed an unimpeachable reputation for scientific objectivity and rationality. However, it severely impaired that reputation in the spring of 1980 with its publication of a booklet called "Toward Healthful Diets." That work raised considerable protest from the American Heart Association and other nutritional authorities because it advised Americans to eat plenty of meat, eggs, butter, and milk despite their high cholesterol content. Investigation of the Board by congressional committee revealed that its members had close affiliations with the meat and dairy interests, wrote their apparently partisan brief without commission from the National Research Council, and were funded by the industry's lobby.

Such questionable procedures cast considerable doubt on the validity of RDA values published by that same Food and Nutrition Board in 1980 (9th edition). Since relatively low RDA estimates obviously benefit the food industry as they make processed products seem nutritionally richer, one must view RDA relevance to your nutritional health with a jaundiced eye.

WHAT ARE THE DANGERS OF VITAMIN "OVERDOSE"?

Vitamins are foods, not drugs, and to speak of vitamin overdosing as if it were comparable to "OD"ing on medications is ridiculous. The possible dangers of getting too much of a drug versus too much of a vitamin are quite different matters. The former can produce permanent injury, even death, while the latter—in the extreme—is equivalent to the discomforts of overeating.

Unregulated enthusiasm for food calories will put on unwanted pounds over months and years, while excessive emphasis on a particular food type, i.e. protein, carbohydrate, or fat, can produce allergic reactions. However, the possibilities of getting too many vitamins are even more remote than the dangers of a too-hearty appetite. For example, the body uses those quantities of C and B-complex vitamins it needs for optimum function and rids itself of any excess within 24 hours—without apparent side effect or injury. Surplus A, D, and E can—after saturating body tissue—produce unpleasant symptoms that disappear when supplementation ceases.[1] However, to achieve such toxicity with fat-soluble vitamins requires consumption of 10 to 20 times the OPA recommendations for A, D, or E every day for months before reaching danger levels. Nonetheless, moderation and caution must be the byword of responsible supplementation. Reduce or eliminate your vitamin regimen at any sign or symptom of distress.

---

1. Toxic levels of the fat-soluble vitamins can produce irreversible damage to the young. Therefore, greatest caution must be exercised in the use of supplementary A, D, or E prior to full maturity and adulthood—i.e. among infants, children, and adolescents.

SHOULD I TAKE MY VITAMINS
AND MINERALS TOGETHER?

Many people—biochemists, dietitians, and physicians as well as laymen—tend to think of vitamins and minerals as nutritional "carts and horses," which is reasonable. They are both dietary essentials required in relatively small quantities when compared with such caloric nutrients as protein, carbohydrate, and fat; they play important roles as co-enzymes in every living cell; and they lead to specific illness when in short supply. Yet there are important differences between these chemical cousins. Unlike vitamins minerals easily survive extremes of chemical and physical processing, are obtained from drinking water as well as foods, and can easily accumulate in the body to cause severe poisoning. For this reason you are probably wise to adhere closely to estimated daily requirements and U.S. RDAs for minerals—unless otherwise directed by a qualified medical practitioner (see Appendix A).

Despite their metabolic differences and because of their metabolic similarities, there is good biochemical reason for taking many vitamins and minerals together in supplement form. For example, vitamins often work more efficiently in the presence of specific minerals, e.g. B_6 with magnesium, pantothenic acid with calcium, E with selenium and manganese. However, not all vitamin-mineral linkages are advantageous, e.g. vitamin E should not be taken at the same time of day as iron. Some minerals deplete your supplies of certain vitamins; e.g. the metabolism of iron requires vitamin C. (For this reason iron supplements for women often contain additional C to protect their body's supply of the vitamin.) Despite these exceptions it is a good general rule to take your vitamins and minerals together—preferably at mealtimes.

I'VE HEARD IT SAID THAT AMERICANS WHO TAKE SUPPLEMENTS HAVE THE RICHEST URINE IN THE WORLD BECAUSE MOST OF THEIR EXPENSIVE VITAMINS PASS RIGHT THROUGH THEIR SYSTEMS. IS THIS TRUE?

Could be a fiscal truth or a fiscal falsehood depending on

how you do your nutritional bookkeeping. We know that the body in its biological wisdom absorbs only those quantities of water-soluble vitamins it needs for optimum function. Any excess is rapidly excreted through the kidneys and bladder without apparent side effect. However, deficiency in these nutrients does not produce such a benign result; the body will cannibalize itself, destroying some of its own cells, to release essential vitamin C and members of the B complex for vital life functions. If you provide your system with more than enough of these vitamins, some will surely be yours on short-term loan. The pennies you spend to ensure a nutritional surplus may pay enormous dividends as you avoid the possibility of the persistent—albeit marginal—vitamin deficiencies that may be linked to chronic, degenerative disease.

MY PHARMACIST TELLS ME THAT THE SUPPLEMENTARY MINERALS I TAKE SHOULD BE "CHELATED." WHY?

Most of the minerals required by your body, e.g. iron, calcium, magnesium, zinc, etc. have a tiny electric charge when dissolved in fluids of the digestive tract. Their charge, which is positive, is identical to that of the membranes lining the small intestine. Since like electrical charges tend to repel, a significant proportion of the minerals taken by mouth may never cross the intestinal divide into the bloodstream. Chelation avoids this problem by surrounding required minerals with a protein coat that reverses their overall electric charge. Since unlike charges attract, the movement of negatively charged chelated minerals through the positively charged intestinal membrane is actually enhanced. By using chelated supplements you can be more certain that your body is actually getting the mineral concentrations you intend.

SHOULD I PAY MORE FOR "NATURAL SOURCE" VITAMINS?

Only if you are convinced that such supplements are nutritionally superior to their manufactured cousins and that they haven't been subjected to the very chemical and physical processing you seek to avoid in buying such a product. Vitamins A and D from "natural source" fish oils or B complex derived from dried liver or yeast can arguably fulfill your expectations of greater nutritional effectiveness and exonerate their additional cost.

MY DOCTOR WANTS ME TO LOSE 20 POUNDS AND HAS ME FOLLOWING A 1,000-CALORIE-A-DAY DIET. HE SUGGESTED I TAKE A VITAMIN/MINERAL SUPPLEMENT EVERY DAY, WHICH SURPRISES ME BECAUSE HE ALWAYS SCOFFED WHEN I SUGGESTED TAKING ONE BEFORE.

Score one for your physician. He is keeping up with latest findings on the health/nutrition front. According to the U.S. Department of Agriculture, many adults—including most women between 23 and 50 years of age—regularly consume 1,500 calories a day or less. Department nutritionists warn that it is virtually impossible to design a diet of less than 2,000 daily calories that will meet even RDA requirements for all vitamins and minerals. Therefore, your weight-loss regimen will almost certainly leave you vitamin deficient and clearly demands supplementation.

I TAKE PRESCRIPTION MEDICATIONS EVERY DAY. CAN I SAFELY TAKE VITAMINS, TOO? SHOULD I TELL MY DOCTOR?

Certainly, to both questions. The regular use of drugs—whether prescription, over-the-counter, or recreational—is apt to elevate your personal vitamin requirements. For example, women on the "pill" have an increased need for the B vitamins—particularly B_6 and folic acid; diuretics—often prescribed to reduce blood pressure or promote weight loss—similarly raise your requirements as they accelerate the flushing of water-soluble vitamins and minerals. Some vitamins—notably C—can improve drug function and help achieve therapeutic effectiveness at lower dosage levels than normally recommended by standard reference works. This is a factor of considerable significance to arthritics using large quantities of aspirin, and diabetics taking insulin. Certain lab tests will give unexpected results if you are following a regimen of supplementation.

In short, tell your physician the exact details of your vitamin program. Be sure to ask if any new medication will alter your nutritional requirements or if a lab procedure can be affected by your supplementation. (See Appendix A for a more complete listing of vitamin/drug interactions.)

A FRIEND TOLD ME THAT VITAMIN C CAN CAUSE KIDNEY STONES. IS THAT TRUE?

If urine becomes excessively acidic, normally liquid waste products from the liver may solidify in the kidneys to form "stones" or "calculi." Such phenomena are relatively rare and usually occur in people with an inherited abnormality in body chemistry.

Because vitamin C is thought of automatically as ascorbic *acid* by many individuals—including physicians—it is assumed that by taking large quantities of ascorbic acid you will acidify your urine and cause kidney stones to form. Such reasoning overlooks the fact that vitamin C in ascorbic acid form undergoes chemical modification before reaching the kidneys and subsequently does little to alter the acid levels of urine.

If you are concerned—possibly because of a family history of kidney disease—use non-acidifying calcium or potassium ascorbate as your source for C.

MY PHYSICIAN TELLS ME TO GET ALL THE VITAMINS I NEED WITH MY KNIFE AND FORK. IS HE RIGHT? CAN I DO IT?

Certainly! if you asked in 1910. Probably! if you asked in 1950. Doubtful! if you ask today. Profound changes in the way we grow, process, market, and prepare our foods have made it increasingly difficult—if not impossible—to get optimal quantities of all the vitamins we need at the dining table. Gone forever are the days when local farmers raised livestock without growth hormones and antibiotics; when they grew their produce without pesticides; and when they could speed genuinely fresh meat, vegetables, and dairy products to your doorstep within hours of milking, harvest, and slaughter.

The newer agribusiness technologies, which have largely replaced the small farm and general store, are awesome. They have created the modern American supermarket that offers an unprecedented array of food choices the year round. Apparently confirming this modern nutritional abundance is the country's bulging waistline, with more than half the adult population seriously overweight. To assume that we are *both* overfed and overnourished is easy. To understand that we are undeniably overfed (with calories) but underfed (with vitamins) has been harder for our health care officials—let alone personal physicians—to understand. Not until 1980 did the U.S. Department of Agriculture publicly recognize the fact that the 1,500-calorie-a-day diet followed by many men and most women to keep their weight in line prevents them from getting even RDA quantities of many vitamins. Thus, officially sanctioned and recommended supplementation has become a very real possibility. Yet the wisdom of your physician's advice—whether 1910, 1950, or in the 1980s—cannot be denied. Vitamin supplements cannot be relied upon to entirely compensate for a poor or indifferent diet. Your pursuit of a calorically balanced menu of nutritionally whole foods must be a primary goal for attaining and preserving good health.

CAN I BELIEVE THAT I'LL ACTUALLY GET THE VITAMIN QUANTITIES OR U.S. RDA PERCENTAGES PRINTED ON FOOD LABELS?

Generally speaking, the answer is affirmative so long as the product is eaten both fresh and uncooked. However, once a processed food product is unsealed, vitamin deterioration begins immediately. Its extent will depend upon length and degree of exposure to heat, light, and air. Because even the best of cooking techniques reduces the vitamin content of food by 50 percent, you can be certain of getting no more than one third to one half of the concentrations indicated on labeled foods that you must cook before eating. (Even bread loses significant quantities of its labeled vitamins when toasted.)

MY VITAMIN SALESMAN TOLD ME THAT WATER-SOLUBLE VITAMINS ARE RAPIDLY ELIMINATED FROM THE BODY AND THAT I WOULD BE WISE TO BUY TIMED-RELEASE SUPPLEMENTS TO BE USED TWO OR THREE TIMES A DAY. THE IDEA SEEMS TO MAKE SENSE. DOES IT?

Your salesman is right up to a point. Blood levels of water-soluble C and B-complex vitamins reach a peak in about 2 hours and fall off rapidly after that. However, it is the vitamin concentration in tissues that is of importance rather than that in the blood. It is inside those tiny microscopic units called cells that the business of life is transacted. Although they absorb their optimum vitamin requirements from the blood very quickly, cells do not break down or release their vitamins or vitamin by-products as rapidly as the circulatory system rids itself of unused vitamins. Achieving vitamin saturation of the blood with water-soluble C and B complex once a day is probably enough to ensure ample supplies of cellular vitamins for any 24-hour period. Thus, the desirability of timed-release supplements may be questioned.

MANY OF MY FRIENDS HAVE BEEN RAVING ABOUT THE WONDERS OF LECITHIN. WHAT IS IT? SHOULD I TAKE IT AS A SUPPLEMENT?

Beware of anyone who "raves" about the miracle properties of any vitamin or mineral. A healthy grain of salt won't cause hardening of the arteries and may protect you against nutritional foolishness. This warning is not meant to downgrade the importance of lecithin in human metabolism nor its possible significance in personal nutrition. However, as with cholesterol, there is little relationship between dietary levels and quantities in the bloodstream —where it counts. Whether you consume lecithin in ordinary foods or in supplement form, it is broken down into its components and loses its chemical identity before absorption across the intestinal wall. It is the liver—the body's biochemical clearinghouse—that ultimately determines how much lecithin will be formed for use by your body, using raw materials derived from the many kinds of fat in your diet (including those contributed by the digestion of dietary lecithin). The amounts synthesized correspond directly with the amount of cholesterol circulating in the blood and undeniably help to prevent the solidification of triglycerides and cholesterol along veins and arteries.

Lecithin's capacity to keep cholesterol and triglycerides from forming blood clots has often been cited as reason for adding lecithin to our diets—as a natural blood-thinning agent. Because the lecithin in your bloodstream has little to do with the lecithin in your diet, its usefulness as a clot preventive is questionable. That it provides an excellent source for choline, a recognized B vitamin, and inositol, a contested B vitamin, is not to be argued. Adding it to your supplement regimen cannot hurt. It may help for as yet poorly understood reasons.

I'VE BEEN SEEING SPECIAL VITAMINS FOR STRESS, SEX, DIETERS, JOGGERS, THINKERS, *ET AL.* ARE THESE PRODUCTS FOR ME?

A 110-pound, 23-year-old female "runner" who does 3 or 4 laps around a city block once or twice a week obviously has quite different vitamin needs from the 185-pound, 55-year-old executive who does 5 miles a day come hell or high water. Although the idea of personalized vitamin regimens is a good one, simply identifying yourself as a "thinker, dieter, or athlete" obviously doesn't provide precise enough information about your biochemical individuality or specific vitamin requirements. (See "Your Personal Vitamin Planner," page 234, for help in developing an individualized program of supplementation.)

ALTHOUGH I'M NOT REALLY SICK VERY OFTEN, I REGULARLY FEEL RUN-DOWN AND LISTLESS, AND HAVE NO OOMPH. MY DOCTOR HAS EXAMINED ME FROM HEAD TO TOE BUT CAN FIND NOTHING PHYSICALLY WRONG WITH ME. COULD VITAMINS HELP?

If your diet is typically calorie rich and vitamin poor, you are probably providing your metabolic machinery with more than enough of the energy fuels it needs but insufficient or inappropriate quantities of the vitamins it requires to properly process those fuels and release the energy locked into their chemical bonds. Such imbalance may be making you quite energy-inefficient, metabolically sluggish, and overweight. By correcting the calorie/vitamin imbalance, your metabolism will potentially release food energy more rapidly and effectively with the result that you feel more of that desired oomph and vitality.

THE LAST TIME I WENT TO MY DENTIST, HE PUT SOME BLUE DROPS UNDER MY TONGUE AND TOLD ME HE WAS MEASURING THE VITAMIN C CONCENTRATION IN MY GUMS. WHAT HAS VITAMIN C GOT TO DO WITH MY TEETH?

There is impressive evidence that the health of gums is often linked to vitamin C concentrations in that tissue. Patients "at saturation" are reported to recover more rapidly from oral surgery and infection, apparently because their levels of C are at maximum. Indeed, many dentists successfully use the vitamin to heal bleeding gums—a condition that often leads to loss of teeth—thereby avoiding the need for painful and expensive periodontal work. The under-the-tongue (sublingual) test used by your dentist is a new, quick, and inexpensive means for determining whether you need additional C to prepare for surgery or to correct a long-standing deficiency that may be a contributing factor to dental problems.

ARE VITAMINS THAT ARE SOLD DOOR-TO-DOOR A GOOD BUY? THEY SEEM TO COST MORE THAN MAIL-ORDER SUPPLEMENTS OR THOSE IN DRUGSTORES.

The answer obviously depends on you, your pocketbook, and the company selling such products. Many of the supplements available from door-to-door salespeople are of a very high quality. Naturally, you must expect to pay a premium for such personalized service. To protect against unnecessary expense, you are wise to pre-plan your vitamin purchases and determine comparative values by investigating the prices of *comparable* products from drugstores, health food outlets, mail-order catalogues, and your door-to-door salesperson.

ARE THERE RELIABLE MEDICAL TESTS TO TELL ME IF I HAVE ANY VITAMIN OR MINERAL DEFICIENCIES?

Until the spring of 1980 it took an average of 4 weeks to measure blood levels of vitamins. A new test that cuts waiting time to 2 days has been developed by research scientists at the New Jersey Medical School. The test must be ordered by your physician and costs $75. Determination of your mineral status can be made through hair analysis conducted by licensed laboratories. Most reliable results are obtained through those laboratories that will only accept samples from your physician and that report their results back to him or her. (See Appendix A for details.)

HOW CAN I FIND A NUTRITIONALLY ORIENTED PHYSICIAN?

It is not easy since fewer than 1 percent of the 300,000 licensed physicians in the United States profess to taking a nutritional approach to medical problems. However, the percentages are growing as increasing numbers of doctors embrace the idea of "holistic medicine"—seeking to prevent as well as to cure disease by employing techniques far beyond those of prescription pad and scalpel. (See Appendix A for directories listing nutritionally oriented practitioners.)

WE HAVE A NUMBER OF FRIENDS WHO REGULARLY TAKE VITAMIN C AND A B-COMPLEX CAPSULE BEFORE GOING TO COCKTAIL PARTIES. HAVE THEY BECOME HEALTH-FOOD NUTS?

The fact that they go to cocktail parties suggests that your friends are still socially, nutritionally, and environmentally mainstream. However, their precautionary use of vitamins is typical of a growing number of health-savvy Americans. Alcohol is a vitamin thief that requires large quantities of the B vitamins—particularly thiamin, or B_1—for its metabolism. If "the Bs" aren't available in the snacks consumed along with drinks, the body will destroy some of its own cells (particularly cells of the liver) to get enough thiamin and the other B vitamins to cope with the booze.

Even if your friends don't smoke, they clearly know that cigarettes go hand-in-hand with cocktails and that they are apt to face a barrage of fumes that will invade their lungs and circulatory systems. Since a single cigarette consumes about 25 mg. of vitamin C, theirs is a wise precaution. It will not provide total immunity against the ravages of cocktails and cigarettes, but it will help to protect sensitive tissue against those poisons.

CAN I GET ALL THE VITAMINS I NEED WITH MY BREAKFAST CEREAL?

The word "need" is at the nub of your question. If you mean "Can my cereal give me the quantities of vitamins and minerals adequate to prevent such depletion diseases as scurvy, beri beri, rickets, or pellagra?"—the answer is a probable "yes" . . . but at an exorbitant price. The nickel's worth of enrichment vitamins added to cereals boasting *total* RDA fulfillment adds an average of 60 cents to their price tag. If your question means "Can I get my optimal personal vitamin allowance with my bowl of breakfast gruel?"—the answer is a probable "no" . . . and you *are* apt to get far more refined sugar than is nutritionally wise. (Up to 50% of some brand-name products is pure sucrose.)

DO I NEED THE SAME QUANTITIES OF VITAMINS EVERY DAY?

Your body's need varies in response to the demands placed upon it. Basic and relatively stable vitamin requirements are personally determined by such factors as inherited biochemistry, age, sex, metabolic rate, and body weight. More variable influences that tend to increase or decrease need in proportion to their relative presence or absence include tension, anxiety, illness, injury, physical activity, use of drugs, exposure to pollutants, and degree of such personal habits as smoking, caffeine consumption, alcohol intake, etc. Unfortunately, we do not possess the kind of vitamin thermometer or blood pressure cuff that could—in theory—tell us our vitamin needs and status in the same way we can quickly check up on our body temperature or blood flow. Therefore, because daily vitamin needs *do vary,* it is wise to aim for levels of supplementation that provide a margin of safety.

I SMOKE MARIJUANA OCCASIONALLY AND USE OTHER RECREATIONAL DRUGS. WHAT WILL BE THE EFFECT ON MY VITAMIN REQUIREMENTS?

Your liver must last a lifetime. Smoking pot or using hard drugs increases its biochemical burden by demanding greater activity from the enzymes that must detoxify the poisons you add to your system. The effect is to increase your personal need for all vitamins—particularly water-soluble C and members of the B complex. Because many drugs irritate the sensitive membranes lining the nose, throat, lung, and digestive tract, your use of such substances also elevates your body's demand for vitamin A. As a word of the greatest caution, don't be gulled into the attractive notion that vitamins can or will compensate for the injury done to body tissue by drugs—whether hard or soft.

CAN VITAMINS BECOME ADDICTIVE?

By definition, addictive substances are ones that create an increasing dependence with prolonged use, so that greater quantities are necessary to achieve the same effect as time passes. Vitamin supplements—in direct contrast—seem to be needed in decreasing quantities with the passage of time. This diminishing need is not surprising as bodily health improves and past deficiencies are corrected.

A second criterion for addiction is the symptoms of withdrawal—often uncomfortable or painful—that come when use of a habit-forming substance ceases. Although you will not experience acute withdrawal symptoms if you stop supplementation abruptly, the body must go through a period of biochemical readjustment as it adapts "cold turkey" to a lower level of vitamins. As your body reaches its optimal level of health, gradual reduction in intake should follow—but such nutritional retrenchment ought to occur over a period of weeks or months.

I'M ABOUT TO HAVE A BABY AND HAVE BEEN TAKING VITAMIN SUPPLEMENTS. WHAT ABOUT MY BABY'S DIET AFTER BIRTH?

Your obstetrician should know the exact details of your vitamin program—which will, of course, be the case if he or she recommended additional vitamins in the first place. It is similarly important to inform or remind the nursing/-medical staff of the hospital where you will give birth of your personal or physician-ordered supplementation. Because your unborn child will have grown and developed in a vitamin-rich environment for 9 months, a sudden withdrawal or decrease in nutritional supply can produce symptoms of vitamin starvation—e.g. a "rebound" scurvy if feedings of C are greatly reduced between the womb and the external world.

Should you breast-feed your child, continuing supplementation will probably be ordered by your physician. Although infant formulas are routinely fortified with vitamins, you and your doctor will want to be certain that the postnatal vitamin diet corresponds to that of prenatal development.

WILL VITAMINS HELP MY ARTHRITIS?

Many nutritionally oriented physicians report considerable success in relieving the symptoms of pain and inflammation associated with the various joint disorders known as arthritis. Some have reported startling remission of the disease. None of these therapies has been adequately tested or proved, and all such regimens require the supervision of medically trained and licensed practitioners.

Although it is unwise to attempt the self-treatment of arthritis, your use of supplements to ensure optimum vitamin nutrition cannot be faulted. Consult your physician before beginning any program of supplementation—being sure to remind him or her that vitamin C makes aspirin more effective and that its addition to your diet can lower analgesic dosages necessary to achieve symptomatic relief from pain and tenderness. Because aspirin is acidic and produces some bleeding along the stomach wall in 75 percent of its users, select *ascorbate* forms of C to avoid compounding the acidic effect.

CAN DIABETICS SAFELY TAKE VITAMINS?

Certainly, but as with any chronic medical condition, it is wise to consult with your physician before beginning an aggressive program of supplementation. Because vitamin C and insulin are chemical allies, any large addition of the vitamin to your daily diet can reduce your need for the hormone. Insulin shock is a theoretical risk, so be certain to monitor your use of the vitamin/hormone combination in close consultation with your physician. (Since C and the bioflavonoids play an important role in maintaining the health of capillaries, supplementation with both is probably advisable to help prevent the circulatory-system deterioration that evidently occurs in the diabetic over long periods despite apparently successful management of the condition with insulin alone.)

WHAT VITAMINS SHOULD I BE TAKING IF I'M ON THE "PILL"?

Oral contraceptives are but one factor in the overall equation that determines your personal vitamin requirements. However, use of the "pill" generally increases your need for vitamins B_6, folic acid, C, and E.

BECAUSE I HAVE A STOMACH ULCER, I MUST AVOID ACIDIC FOODS. DOES THIS MEAN I CAN'T TAKE VITAMIN C?

Fortunately, you can forego supplementary acidity without giving up your C. Although ascorbic acid is the most frequent source of the vitamin—whether in citrus fruits or supplements—the *ascorbate* forms (usually calcium or potassium) are non-acidic, widely available, and as biochemically effective as the more familiar ascorbic acid.

NOTE: Switching from ascorbic acid to ascorbate is probably a good idea if C seems to upset your stomach or cause diarrhea.

MY HUSBAND AND I HAVE A BUSY SOCIAL SCHEDULE, WHICH MEANS WE PROBABLY DRINK MORE ALCOHOL IN A WEEK THAN IS GOOD FOR US. CAN VITAMINS BE OF HELP?

Your first goal ought to be eliminating or controlling the poison before seeking an antidote. Although business and social gatherings often seem to demand an alcoholic solvent, there is no reason why you can't substitute a light white wine or mineral water with a twist of lemon for hard liquor on most occasions.

Because alcohol is an almost pure, refined carbohydrate, it is a voracious vitamin thief that demands heavy concentrations of the B vitamins—particularly B_1, or thiamin—and C for its proper chemical processing. Adding a high potency B supplement with C to your daily dietary regimen will help reduce—but not eliminate—the tissue damage resulting from overimbibing.

IT IS VERY DIFFICULT FOR ME TO EAT PROPERLY—YOU KNOW, THREE BALANCED MEALS A DAY. ARE VITAMINS GOOD INSURANCE?

Your coverage will be only partial and hardly reliable because there simply is no substitute for careful attention to the quality and quantity of what you eat. Although a calorically balanced diet drawn from a wide variety of fresh foods will not automatically provide you with optimum quantities of all nutrients, it will increase your chances for good health. Vitamins alone cannot totally compensate for careless eating—e.g. reliance on highly refined and processed foods.

I AM A 45-YEAR-OLD WOMAN GOING THROUGH THE CHANGE OF LIFE WITHOUT TOO MANY PROBLEMS. BECAUSE I HAVE FAIR SKIN THAT DOESN'T TOLERATE THE SUN WITHOUT BURNING AND I CAN'T DRINK MILK, MY DOCTOR WANTS ME TO TAKE A DAILY SUPPLEMENT OF VITAMIN D. WHY? ISN'T THAT DANGEROUS?

First and foremost, these are questions for your doctor. However, he or she is probably concerned about preventing a condition known as *osteoporosis,* which has become increasingly frequent among senior citizens—particularly women. It is associated with long-term, sub-clinical deficiencies of vitamin D that prevent the proper absorption of calcium from the diet. The result is "brittle bones" that fracture easily and are slow to heal.

Because our principal sources of vitamin D are exposure to sunlight (interaction with natural skin oils) and vitamin-fortified milk, your individual—but not uncommon—sensitivities put you "at risk" for osteoporosis. By taking regular supplements of D at this time you may well prevent the disease—which does not respond to the vitamin once actual symptoms of bone brittleness appear. Undoubtably, the quantities of D your physician recommends should pose no danger. The clear and present threat is from getting too little of the vitamin.

I HAVE A TERRIBLE CASE OF ACNE. MY FRIENDS ARE TAKING SUPER QUANTITIES OF VITAMIN A. WHAT DO YOU THINK?

I think your friends are extremely foolish unless their therapy is closely supervised by a physician. While there is considerable evidence that vitamin A and its chemical cousins will help control acne, required concentrations border on amounts that threaten to poison you. Your physician—and only your physician—can *prescribe* alternative forms of A that are considerably less toxic than those you obtain over-the-counter. Furthermore, no one but your doctor can be certain you obtain therapeutic dosages appropriate to your condition and biochemical individuality.

I REGULARLY SUFFER FROM PAINFUL AND IRRITATING COLD SORES. IS IT TRUE THAT NUTRITIONAL SUPPLEMENTS CAN HELP ME?

Various forms of the herpes virus seem to cause these painful lesions along mucous membranes lining the nose, mouth, lips, genitalia, and even the eyes among susceptible individuals. Some seem to be born with the offending virus, others acquire it through sexual contact. Evidently, once infected—by heredity or environment—you are apt to carry the virus for the rest of your life and suffer from periodic flareups of the characteristic sores during periods of stress.

Studies at the Mayo Clinic indicate that the daily use of 312 mg of the amino acid *lysine* helps prevent or suppress the herpes lesion. Other studies recommend the use of lysine in combination with 1 to 2 grams of vitamin C. Because cold sores represent a genuine medical condition (recognized as pre-cancerous when it occurs in the cervix), be sure to consult your physician about its treatment and/-or possible prevention.

MY 8-YEAR-OLD SON IS HYPERACTIVE. WILL VITAMINS HELP?

Hyperactivity is a medical condition that requires a physician's attention and supervision. If he or she proposes standard drug therapies, e.g. the amphetamine called Ritalin, you may properly object since the use of "speed" to control hyperactivity evidently retards proper growth and development in a significant number of children. Furthermore, such treatment simply copes with symptoms rather than causes of the disorder.

Reports linking hyperactivity to diets rich in refined carbohydrates; food additives, dyes, and preservatives; and/or undetected vitamin deficiencies have gained considerable attention in recent years. Your pediatrician may be willing to try a rigorous dietary approach using vitamins, or you may seek the assistance of a nutritionally oriented physician (see Appendix A).

NOTE: It would be foolhardy to attempt to cure your child's hyperactivity using vitamin supplements alone.

CAN I TAKE MY VITAMIN SUPPLEMENTS WITH ME TO THE HOSPITAL?

If you have been taking supplements on a regular basis, it is advisable on a number of counts. Your body becomes adapted to the levels of vitamins you regularly feed it and sudden withdrawal—particularly during the physical stress ordinarily associated with hospitalization—can undermine your system at a time when it must function at its best. Indeed, increasing numbers of surgeons are recommending intensive vitamin supplementation, particularly with C, before and after surgery to promote healing. The same is increasingly true of physicians prescribing drug therapy, as there is growing evidence that aggressive supplementation can lower needed drug dosage and accelerate elimination of toxic drug byproducts from the body (thereby reducing the risk of undesirable side effects).

Whatever the reasons for your hospitalization, it is of utmost importance to inform *all* medical staff—your physician, nurses, lab technicians, and medical residents or interns, who may take your medical history—of past supplementation. Following their recommendations while under their professional care is of utmost importance.

ON READING THE FINE PRINT OF MY SUPPLEMENT LABEL, I SEE IT CONTAINS SUCH SUBSTANCES AS STEARATE, GLYCOL, AND FOOD COLORING BESIDES VITAMINS. DO SUCH CHEMICALS BELONG IN A SUPPLEMENT?

They are certainly not essential to your good health and nutrition. However, the quantities of preservatives, colorants, and emulsifiers in such products is minuscule—particularly in comparison with the amounts you unavoidably consume with your daily diet (unless you are fortunate enough to grow all of your own food). Such substances—even in trace concentrations—can be a cause of upset in susceptible individuals. Try products without such additives if you have trouble tolerating a supplement. The additives, not the vitamins, may be at fault.

CAN VITAMINS HELP MY ALLERGIES?

Possibly! "Allergy" is an umbrella term that describes a wide variety of negative biological responses by your body to its chemical and physical environment. Allergists generally define the disorders they treat as any condition in which specific irritants, e.g. dust, animal dander, pollen, smoke, etc., inappropriately stimulate your body's immune defenses as if they were life-threatening bacterial or viral invaders. A broader definition includes any regular bodily revolt against the chemically hostile intrusion of sensitive tissue from the air we breathe (pollutants), water we drink (impurities), and/or foods we eat (additives). Because detoxification of your chemical enemies depends on specific vitamins, their presence in ample and balanced quantities is an important factor in your biochemical armor; but it is critical to remember that allergies are conditions requiring medical supervision. Be sure to discuss the use of supplements with your allergist and on no account attempt vitamin self-treatment of your allergic sensitivity.

I'VE HEARD THERE ARE MANY DIFFERENT KINDS OF VITAMINS A, D, AND E. DO THEY MATTER OR ARE THEY JUST ANOTHER WAY TO GET ME TO SPEND MORE MONEY FOR SUPPLEMENTS?

Pure vitamin A, or retinol, is generally included in supplements derived from fish oils and dissolved in fat, or it may be chemically combined with acetate or palmitate to allow it to disperse in water. The latter form is recommended for anyone intolerant of oil, e.g. acne sufferers. Provitamin A, or B-carotene, is often included in "natural" products extracted from vegetable sources. Our bodies normally convert B-carotene into vitamin A without difficulty. However, this transformation of the provitamin into usable A may not take place if you regularly use mineral oil or have difficulty absorbing nutrients from your digestive tract. Oil-based retinol or its water-based acetate or palmitate equivalent is probably your safer choice.

The vitamin D derived from animal sources, e.g. fish oil, is called cholecalciferol, or D_3; that extracted from plant tissue is known as ergocalciferol, or D_2. Both forms of the vitamin have about the same degree of biochemical activity, although supplements containing D_3 may be marginally more effective in human metabolism. Products delivering other forms of vitamin D are biologically inferior.

There are at least 8 different varieties of vitamin E. All are known as tocopherols. Far and away the most potent is alpha (α) tocopherol. Supplements usually contain alpha-tocopherol alone, or alpha-tocopherol and "mixed tocopherols." The nutritional effectiveness of mixed tocopherols has not been demonstrated.

EVERYONE KNOWS THAT THE DOLOMITES ARE MOUN-
TAINS IN EUROPE. WOULD YOU BELIEVE THAT SOME
QUACK IS NOW BOTTLING A GRAY POWDER THAT LOOKS
LIKE FINE GRAVEL, CALLING IT DOLOMITE, AND SUG-
GESTING THAT PEOPLE SHOULD TAKE SOME EVERY DAY?

Your knowledge of geography rates an "A", but your
familiarity with mineral nutrition is a "pure flunk." Dolomite is a mixture of calcium and magnesium—2 minerals
essential to human metabolism. The ratio of twice as much
calcium as magnesium in dolomite corresponds to the
desired balance in your body. Because most dietary calcium (milk, cheese, and other dairy products) depends on
vitamin D for absorption, the fact that calcium in dolomite doesn't require D to be put to use makes it a doubly
attractive supplement—particularly for the many adults
who get little sun and can't tolerate vitamin D–enriched
milk. Supplementation with dolomite should provide you
with about 800 mg of calcium and 400 mg of magnesium
per day.

MY PHYSICIAN SAYS THERE IS NO SCIENTIFIC PROOF
THAT VITAMIN SUPPLEMENTS DO ANY GOOD. IS THAT
TRUE?

Astonishing! Vitamins are important and recognized medical tools routinely used by physicians for the treatment of
a wide range of disorders including many varieties of anemia, eye diseases, circulatory problems, and digestive difficulties to name but a few. So, to begin with, his or her
assertion must refer only to the regular use of supplements
as a preventive among apparently healthy individuals.

According to the FDA there are two criteria by
which a substance is to be scientifically judged—its comparative safety and its effectiveness.

With 75 million Americans using supplements on a
daily basis, there is ample proof of safety. No one has died
from oversupplementation, while documented cases of injury are extremely rare and generally involve the enormously exaggerated intake of fat-soluble vitamin A over
long periods of time.

Although effectiveness is more difficult to prove when the question is one of prevention rather than cure, even the most ardent critics now agree that vitamin C does reduce the severity of cold symptoms among significant numbers of people. (See Appendix B for further evidence of vitamin effectiveness.)

I'M 60 YEARS OLD AND HAVE HEART DISEASE. MANY OF MY FRIENDS WITH SIMILAR PROBLEMS ARE FOLLOWING WELL-KNOWN DIETS THAT ARE INTENDED TO HELP PREVENT HEART ATTACK AND STROKE. MOST RECOMMEND PROGRAMS OF VITAMIN SUPPLEMENTATION. OTHERS DON'T. WHAT'S THE LATEST EVIDENCE?

Although the American Heart Association has for many years linked heart disease to diet—particularly to high levels of blood cholesterol—it and other medical authorities are skeptical about the effectiveness of the widely publicized diet plans of which you speak. Criticism is officially based on the absence of hard and fast statistics to prove or disprove the effectiveness of such diets. Nonetheless, most such regimens incorporate sound nutritional thinking and prudent practices. Those that recommend vitamin supplementation do so because of increasing evidence that links the health of heart muscle and circulatory conduits to optimum vitamin nutrition. (See Appendix B for a more detailed discussion.) The one program that discourages the use of supplements is also the most stringent—relying entirely on draconian dietary measures that seek to obtain optimum vitamin intake through unprocessed, vitamin-rich foods. Significant problems with the diet include its expense, the difficulty of obtaining such vitamin-rich ingredients, and a strong psychological sense of deprivation that accompanies a lifetime commitment to so restricted a menu.

Your concern about diet and your condition is wise. Personal reading and research—along with close physician consultation—should help you make the nutritional choices best and most tolerable to you. Vitamins will play an important role in your regimen, whether from natural food sources or from supplements.

MY MEMORY IS SLIPPING. I'VE HEARD THAT VITAMINS CAN HELP. IS THERE ANY TRUTH TO THE RUMOR?

The transmission of nerve impulses—including those in the brain associated with memory—are dependent upon a substance called *acetylcholine.* The body's synthesis of the compound depends directly on dietary supplies of the B vitamin *choline.* Research begun at the Massachusetts Institute of Technology (MIT) in 1975 has increasingly linked choline insufficiency with memory impairment, particularly among senior citizens.

The findings are significant because as many as 15 percent of those over 65 suffer from Alzheimer's disease, a relentless illness that typically begins with memory loss and tends to develop over 5 to 10 years into full-blown dementia or senility. The use of supplementary choline, lecithin (containing choline), or a diet rich in meat and eggs evidently helps prevent or slow the course of this disease.

Similar supplementation apparently allays the powerful side effects of anti-psychotic drugs that inhibit the release of choline in the brain and produce a bizarre condition, *tardive dyskinesia,* in which patients develop uncontrolled twitching movements, facial grimacing, and spasms of the tongue.

I SPEND CLOSE TO $15 A MONTH ON VITAMIN SUPPLEMENTS FOR MY HUSBAND AND MYSELF. THAT SEEMS LIKE A LOT OF MONEY.

The country's per capita spending for food and medical care is about 20 times that amount every 30 days. Of course, you are not "average" (since "Jane and John Doe" are convenient statistical myths) so your actual contribution to health insurance plans, your physician's pocketbook, and the supermarket cash register may vary considerably from the national average. However, the kinds of advantages you may enjoy for $7.50 per person per month probably make yours an excellent investment. If—for a single example—the vitamin C you take reduces the severity of cold symptoms and days lost from productive work by the 50% even most ardent critics of the vitamin agree upon, your health and fiscal returns are enormous.

WHY DO SO MANY FAMOUS AND EVIDENTLY INTELLIGENT PEOPLE GO TO VITAMIN "QUACKS" IF THEY HAVE CANCER?

The reasons are many and by no means universal, but it is a sad fact that in many such widely publicized cases the celebrity in question has followed all of the traditional medical treatments, which have ultimately failed to arrest his or her disease. It is an unfortunate but documented truth that the attitude of medical-care professionals toward terminally ill cancer patients often undergoes a subtle but insidious change. The patient over whom they have struggled and lost is apt to be viewed as a defeat, and the kind of strong emotional support so desperately needed by the dying is often withdrawn at the most crucial moment. As human hope springs eternal, even against the most formidable odds, it is not surprising that the terminally ill patient will turn to any alternative therapy that will offer hope or at least active resistance to death. Unfortunately, such thoroughly advanced cases are often beyond any kind of medical/nutritional help and the patients thus appear to have died at the hands of a "quack."

DIETARY RECOMMENDATIONS FROM THE "AUTHORITIES" ARE VERY CONFUSING. HOW CAN ONE EAT SENSIBLY?

Confusion about nutrition abounds—as much among establishment "experts" as the general public. Failure to take the role of diet seriously in human health has been a besetting sin of American science and medicine. Assuming that because we are calorically overfed we must inevitably be overnourished has been an easy assumption that keeps the research community from establishing a rigorous nutritional science. All that authority figures seem to agree on is the wisdom of "eating a balanced diet, drawing on a wide variety of foods from the various food groups." This recipe for nutritional good health is hardly scientific or particularly useful. Witness the trained dietitians and nutritionists who have followed the formulation by feeding hospital patients a "balanced" menu of canned and frozen, overcooked foods from the various food categories. Who can really be surprised that studies of hospitalized patients reveal a shocking incidence of malnourishment that often undermines recovery from surgery or infection? Referring to pie-shaped graphs that tell us our diets should be X percent protein, Y percent carbohydrate, and Z percent fat isn't much help either.

In the absence of a rigorous nutritional science, personal good sense must prevail. Prudent eating must keep you from becoming overweight or obese. Choosing genuinely fresh foods in the place of highly processed alternatives is a clear desideratum. Whole-grained, complex carbohydrates are clearly preferable to simple sugars; fats—whether saturated or unsaturated—need to be restricted; protein from vegetable sources or the lean white meat of poultry or fish is probably better for you than that of red meat. Overcooking destroys valuable nutrients. Such simple-minded nutritional rules don't offer much, but they are a beginning.

Appendix D

Personal Vitamin Planner

YOUR SUPPLEMENT PROGRAM

Formulating a vitamin regimen tailored to your biochemical needs and nutritional philosophy is essential—before shopping for supplement products. If you choose a program conforming to U.S. RDA standards, be sure to consult the appropriate chart (pages 78–79). If you intend to pursue a more aggressive program, be certain to reread Chapter 5 and estimate your need for each vitamin using the OPA guidelines (pages 154–155)—before planning your personal supplement program, below.

	U.S. RDA Program	OPA Program
Vitamins		
Fat Soluble:		
Vit. A	_____ IU	_____ IU
Vit. D	_____ IU	_____ IU
Vit. E	_____ IU	_____ IU

	U.S. RDA	OPA
Vitamins		
Water Soluble:		
Vit. C	_____ mg/g	_____ mg/g
B Complex:		
Folic Acid, FA	_____ mcg/mg	_____ mcg/mg
Thiamin, B_1	_____ mg	_____ mg
Riboflavin, B_2	_____ mg	_____ mg
Niacin, B_3	_____ mg	_____ mg
Pyridoxine, B_6	_____ mg	_____ mg
Cobalamin, B_{12}	_____ mcg/mg	_____ mcg/mg
Biotin	_____ mcg	_____ mcg
Panto. Acid	_____ mg	_____ mg
Contested:		
Inositol	x	_____ mg
PABA	x	_____ mg
Pangamate,[1] B_{15}	x	_____ mg
Bioflavonoids	x	_____ mg

		OPA
Minerals (Optional)		
Recognized/U.S. RDAs:	U.S.RDA	(U.S. RDA)[2]
Calcium, Ca	_____ mg	_____ mg
Phosphorus, P	_____ mg	_____ mg
Iodine, I	_____ mcg/mg	_____ mcg/mg
Iron, Fe	_____ mg	_____ mg
Magnesium, Mg	_____ mg	_____ mg
Copper, Cu	_____ mg	_____ mg
Zinc, Zn	_____ mg	_____ mg
Recognized/No U.S. RDAs:		OPAs (RDAs)[3]
Chromium, Cr	x	_____ mg
Cobalt, Co	x	x
Lithium, Li	x	x
Manganese, Mn	x	_____ mg
Molybdenum, Mb	x	_____ mg
Selenium, Se	x	_____ mg
Vanadium, Vn	x	x

1. N,N-Dimethylglycine.   2. Values are the same.
3. See Table, page 244. Co, Li, and Vn have no estimated OPA (RDA) value.

NOTES

Once you have determined your ideal vitamin/mineral program, it is possible to select products that will fit your personal needs and pocketbook.

a. Single-capsule or -tablet formulations that contain all officially recognized vitamins and minerals in U.S. RDA quantities are widely available. Selection among them should be based on considerations of price, ease of consumption, nature of the binders/fillers, and whether their "extraction from natural sources" or synthesis from scratch is of importance to you.

b. To fulfill the requirements of more aggressive supplementation programs usually requires a combination of products. Beginning with a basic multiple that contains all or most of your required vitamins, you can meet your unique needs by the addition of single-ingredient supplements. For example—

Vitamin	Your OPA Program	A Typical High-Potency Product
A	5,000 IU	5,000 IU
D	400 IU	400 IU
E	100 IU	100 IU
C	2,000 mg (2 g)	500 mg (½ g)
FA	500 mcg	100 mcg
B_1	50 mg	50 mg
B_2	50 mg	50 mg
B_3	100 mg	100 mg
B_6	50 mg	50 mg
B_{12}	50 mcg	50 mcg
Biotin	50 mcg	50 mcg
Panto. Acid	150 mg	50 mg

To complete your regimen you will need to add daily single supplements of C (1,500 mg or 1½ g), FA (400 mcg), and panto. acid (100 mg)—all readily available in the marketplace.

This is but one way to "skin the cat" to fulfill your OPA program. There are many others that depend upon personal need and choice; for example, because of size limitations, multiple-vitamin products derived from organic sources often do not approach desired supplementation levels in a single capsule or tablet. However, taking 1 or 2 with each of 3 daily meals often will bring you to your appropriate daily quota while ensuring steady-state blood concentrations over a 24-hour period. Similarly, you might choose 3 separate products: one containing all the fat-soluble vitamins for use every day or every other day; a second containing 500 mg to 1,000 mg (1 g) of C to be taken once or more daily; and a third balanced B-50, B-75, or B-100. The possible combinations are enormous and a matter of individual preference; even the consumption of separate, single-ingredient products—which is expensive and a great deal to swallow.

c. Many supplements include various quantities of the recognized minerals essential for good health. Unlike vitamins, these nutrients generally survive agribusiness processing, are acquired from non-nutritional sources as well as food—e.g. drinking water—and can be highly toxic in excessive concentrations. Supplementation beyond U.S. RDAs cannot be recommended unless you undergo the kinds of medical testing described in Appendix A. Mineral deficiencies *are* increasingly implicated in the occurrence of both infectious and degenerative disorders. Their correction requires careful monitoring by a nutritionally oriented physician (also Appendix A).

d. Trace minerals necessary for life but currently lacking U.S. RDAs are often present in supplement products. They include chromium, Cr; cobalt, Co; lithium, Li; manganese, Mn; molybdenum, Mo; selenium, Se; and vanadium, Vn. Deficiency states for these elements are associated with developing or outright disease but they shouldn't be consumed in excess of RDA estimated values (see page 244) without laboratory analyses to determine your unique status for each.

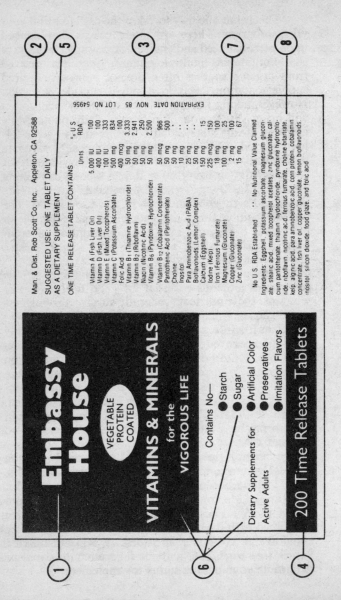

Man. & Dist. Rob Scott Co. Inc. Appleton. CA 92588

EXPIRATION DATE NOV 85 LOT NO 54956

SUGGESTED USE: ONE TABLET DAILY
AS A DIETARY SUPPLEMENT

ONE TIME RELEASE TABLET CONTAINS

	Units	% U.S. RDA
Vitamin A (Fish Liver Oil)	5,000 IU	100
Vitamin D (Fish Liver Oil)	400 IU	100
Vitamin E (Mixed Tocopherols)	100 IU	333
Vitamin C (Potassium Ascorbate)	500 mg	834
Folic Acid	400 mcg	100
Vitamin B₁ (Thiamine Hydrochloride)	50 mg	3,333
Vitamin B₂ (Riboflavin)	50 mg	2,941
Niacin (Nicotinic Acid)	50 mg	250
Vitamin B6 (Pyridoxine Hydrochloride)	50 mg	2,500
Vitamin B12 (Cobalamin Concentrate)	50 mcg	966
Pantothenic Acid (Pantothenate)	50 mg	500
Choline	50 mg	··
Inositol	10 mg	··
Para Aminobenzoic Acid (PABA)	25 mg	··
Bioflavonoids (Lemon Complex)	50 mg	··
Calcium (Eggshell)	150 mg	15
Iodine (Kelp)	225 mcg	150
Iron (Ferrous Fumarate)	18 mg	100
Magnesium (Gluconate)	100 mg	25
Copper (Gluconate)	2 mg	100
Zinc (Gluconate)	15 mg	67

No U.S. RDA Established   ·· No Nutritional Value Claimed

Ingredients: Eggshell, potassium ascorbate, magnesium gluconate, stearic acid, mixed tocopherol acetates, zinc gluconate, calcium pantothenate, thiamin hydrochloride, pyridoxine hydrochloride, riboflavin, nicotinic acid, ferrous fumarate, choline bitartrate, kelp, alginic acid, para aminobenzoic acid, corn protein, cobalamin concentrate, fish liver oil, copper gluconate, lemon bioflavonoids, inositol, silicon dioxide, food glaze, and folic acid.

Embassy House

VEGETABLE PROTEIN COATED

VITAMINS & MINERALS
for the
VIGOROUS LIFE

Contains No—
● Starch
● Sugar
● Artificial Color
● Preservatives
● Imitation Flavors

Dietary Supplements for Active Adults

200 Time Release Tablets

HOW TO READ A SUPPLEMENT LABEL

An Informative Label: What to Look For

The amount of information appearing on the label of a vitamin product is apt to be enormous—particularly for a multivitamin/multimineral supplement. The data a manufacturer must supply by law and wishes to include for promotional purposes poses a printing problem not dissimilar to that of inscribing the Lord's Prayer on the head of a pin. Confronted by the array of fine print, you may feel you need a magnifying glass for legibility and a chemical dictionary for comprehension. Nonetheless, the time and effort you spend in reading the fine print and asking appropriate questions will correspond to the quality of the product and supplementation you obtain.

NOTES *(See Embassy House label, opposite.)*

1. *Brand Name:* The largest and richest vitamin manufacturers—usually major pharmaceutical houses—annually spend tens of millions of dollars on radio, television, and print advertising. The primary intent is to condition a consumer to identify their trade name as synonymous with the entire category of vitamin supplements; i.e. success is complete when you think of buying your "One-a-Days" or "Stresstabs" instead of simply "vitamins." The considerable cost of such persuasion is generally passed along to the purchaser, who is often happy to settle for a familiar name when faced with the bewildering number of vitamin choices in today's pharmacies, supermarkets, and health food stores. Unfortunately, the recognition of a brand name tells you next to nothing about the quality or appropriateness of the product represented and should have only a marginal impact on your selection of a supplement.

2. *Manufacturer's Name and Address:* Many major vitamin producers sell their supplements to independent
   wholesalers and retailers, who may in turn affix their
   own labels to such trade-name formulations. Some will
   appear in the marketplace as "no brand," generic, or
   mail order supplements that offer you a trade-name
   formulation at reduced rates, while others will appear
   as private-label products at higher, lower, or equivalent
   prices depending upon the retailer. Your clue to the
   origin of an unfamiliar supplement is the producer's or
   distributor's name and address. If you have questions
   about any generic, private-label, or brand-name product, write to the manufacturer. Most have customer
   service departments that are happy to respond to your
   questions. (See Directory of American and Canadian
   Vitamin Manufacturers, page 317).

3. *Date of Expiration/Lot Number:* Vitamins—even in
   supplement form—are fragile substances that can lose
   their potency after a few years of shelflife, even when
   tightly sealed in lightproof containers and packed with
   absorbent cotton or desiccant capsules that control hu-
   midity. The presence of a potency expiration date—
   beyond which a product should be neither bought nor
   used—and the inclusion of a lot number on a supplement is a good sign that the manufacturer is carefully
   monitoring the biochemical quality of his vitamins.
   Lack of such information is sufficient grounds for not
   purchasing a product.

4. *Number of Supplements per Container:* The daily cost
   of supplementation varies enormously. Unfortunately,
   the unit pricing now widely in effect for supermarket
   groceries rarely extends to vitamin products. To determine the cost of a day's supplementation, divide the
   total retail price by the number of tablets, capsules, or
   servings (liquids or drops) in the container. Remember,
   a comprehensive multivitamin/mineral supplement
   that costs twenty-five cents daily may be a better bar-
   gain than the dime-a-day product that requires addi-

tional single-ingredient supplements to meet your personal requirements.

5. *Recommended Consumption/Suggested Use:* These guidelines from the manufacturer are intended to help those without a preplanned regimen of supplementation. Be aware that while most content labels express their vitamin concentrations (IUs, gs, mgs, or mcgs) and U.S. RDA percentages in terms of a single tablet or capsule, others that recommend daily consumption of anywhere from 2 to 6 units normally describe their vitamin/mineral strengths on the assumption that you take a full daily allotment, i.e. 2 to 6 capsules, tablets, or liquid servings. The latter variety of supplement offers you nutritional flexibility but may add considerably to your cost.

6. *Advertising Claims:* Cast a wary eye over this portion of any vitamin label. In the sample label, "Embassy House" wants you to know that its product contains no starch, sugar, preservatives, artificial coloring, or imitation flavorings—useful information to be sure, but negative virtues that say nothing about what the product does contain, i.e. the source of its vitamin and mineral components, which are largely synthesized. That the nutritionally active ingredients are delivered in a timed-release protein-coated tablet is important—but one man's "vigorous life" and notion of an "active adult" is another's boredom and lethargy. Beware the glittering generality and promise of the instant good life.

7. *Contents Panel:* This is the single most important section of any supplement label. Its inclusion is mandated by law and must include in prescribed order all nutritionally active ingredients by name or letter designation (e.g. vitamin A, or retinol; Ca, or calcium); the strength for each nutrient expressed in standard concentrations (IUs, gs, mgs, or mcgs), and the percentage of U.S. RDAs for each. Compare the information on this panel

with your preplanned vitamin program (see page 234) to determine a product's relevancy for you.

The contents panel for "Embassy House" vitamins and minerals includes the following information:

	UNITS	% U.S. RDA
Vitamin A (Fish Liver Oil)	5,000 IU	100
Vitamin D (Fish Liver Oil)	400 IU	100
Vitamin E (Mixed Tocopherols)	100 IU	333
Vitamin C (Potassium Ascorbate)	500 mg	834
Folic Acid	400 mcg	100
Vitamin B$_1$ (Thiamin Hydrochloride)	50 mg	3,333
Vitamin B$_2$ (Riboflavin)	50 mg	2,941
Niacin (Nicotinic Acid)	50 mg	250
Vitamin B$_6$ (Pyridoxine Hydrochloride)	50 mg	2,500
Vitamin B$_{12}$ (Cobalamin Concentrate)	50 mcg	966
Pantothenic Acid (Pantothenate)	50 mg	500
Choline	50 mg	*
Inositol	10 mg	**
Para Aminobenzoic Acid (PABA)	25 mg	**
Bioflavonoids (Lemon Complex)	50 mg	**
Calcium (Eggshell)	150 mg	15
Iodine (Kelp)	225 mcg	150
Iron (Ferrous Fumarate)	18 mg	100
Magnesium (Gluconate)	100 mg	25
Copper (Gluconate)	2 mg	100
Zinc (Gluconate)	15 mg	67

*No U.S. RDA Established
**No Nutritional Value Claimed

You will notice that the product—
a. does not include either *biotin,* a recognized B vitamin, or *phosphorus,* a recognized nutritional mineral —both of which have U.S. RDA values.
b. does include 3 of the contested vitamins (inositol, PABA, and the bioflavonoids) and one recognized vitamin that currently lacks a U.S. RDA (choline).
c. does indicate some—but not all—of the sources for its active ingredients, e.g. vitamins A and D from fish oils, and the chemical form of its contents, e.g. vita-

min C as non-acidic ascorbate rather than ascorbic acid.

d. does not make any claim to be "natural" or "organic," so that you may assume—correctly—that some of its nutrients have been synthesized.

8. *Ingredients List:* New nutritional labeling laws require that food products identify their ingredients in decreasing order of concentration. Thus, a processed cheese may list granular skim milk cheese, whey, skim milk, sodium citrate, cream, salt, sodium phosphate, and sorbic acids as its ingredients. This tells you that granular skim milk cheese is the most concentrated component, while sorbic acid is its least concentrated. The same ordering applies to supplement ingredient lists. In the case of multivitamin/mineral products with many components, cursory examination may alarm you because of the inclusion of many foreign-sounding chemicals. For example, the ingredients panel for "Embassy House" vitamins and minerals includes 25 substances:

Ingredients: Eggshell, potassium *ascorbate, magnesium* gluconate, stearic acid, mixed *tocopherol* acetates, *zinc* gluconate, calcium *pantothenate, thiamin* hydrochloride, *pyridoxine* hydrochloride, *riboflavin, nicotinic acid, ferrous* fumarate, *choline* bitartrate, *kelp,* alginic acid, *para aminobenzoic acid,* corn protein, *cobalamin* concentrate, *fish liver oil, copper* gluconate, lemon *bioflavonoids, inositol,* silicon dioxide, food glaze, and *folic acid*

At first glance the list is truly frightening. It is less so when you realize that most of the ingredient name describes the biochemical delivery form for the desired vitamins and minerals; e.g. vitamin C as potassium *ascorbate,* pantothenic acid from calcium *pantothenate,* copper from copper *gluconate,* etc.[3] The only ingredients not identified with a specific and desired vitamin or

---

3. The Synonyms sections of Chapter 4, "Vitamin Profiles," will help you identify the chemical names of synthesized ingredients. (The italics used here are generally not found on labels.)

mineral are stearic acid, alginic acid, corn protein, silicon dioxide, and food glaze. These are the binders and fillers used to compound the product. They may be important to you if you experience digestive upset while using the supplement, are concerned about "natural" ingredients,[4] or are prone to food additive allergies.

Many vitamin supplement products also contain minerals. Unlike vitamins, minerals generally survive processing, are found in drinking water in varying concentrations, and can be toxic in amounts just a few times as large as those required by your body for proper functioning. Recommended amounts of certain minerals can be found in the RDA and U.S. RDA charts (pages 64–65 and 78–79). The figures in the following charts, based on less than conclusive studies, are provided because these minerals are also included in many supplement products.

Estimated Safe and Adequate Daily Dietary Intakes of Selected Minerals[a]

| | Age (years) | Trace Elements[b] | | | | |
		Chromium (mg)	Copper (mg)	Manganese (mg)	Molybdenum (mg)	Selenium (mg)
Infants	0.0–0.5	0.01–0.04	0.5–0.7	0.5–0.7	0.03–0.06	0.01–0.04
	0.5–1.0	0.02–0.06	0.7–1.0	0.7–1.0	0.04–0.06	0.02–0.06
Children	1–3	0.02–0.08	1.0–1.5	1.0–1.5	0.05–0.1	0.02–0.08
and	4–6	0.03–0.12	1.5–2.0	1.5–2.0	0.06–0.15	0.03–0.12
Adolescents	7–10	0.05–0.2	2.0–2.5	2.0–3.0	0.10–0.3	0.05–0.2
	11+	0.05–0.2	2.0–3.0	2.5–5.0	0.15–0.5	0.05–0.2
Adults		0.05–0.2	2.0–3.0	2.5–5.0	0.15–0.5	0.05–0.2

From *Recommended Dietary Allowances,* Food and Nutrition Board, National Academy of Sciences-National Research Council, 1980.

[a] Because there is less information on which to base allowances, these figures are not given in the main table of RDA and are provided here in the form of ranges of recommended intakes.

[b] Since the toxic levels for many trace elements may be only several times usual intakes, the upper levels for the trace elements given in this table should not be habitually exceeded.

---

4. The Principal Sources sections of Chapter 4, "Vitamin Profiles," will aid in identifying the vitamin forms from natural sources, e.g. B complex derived from yeast or desiccated liver, calcium from eggshells, etc.

Mineral electrolytes—sodium (Na), potassium (K), and chloride (Cl)—are essential for the transmission of nerve impulses and other critical biochemical processes. Table salt (sodium chloride) is the principal source of supply for Na and Cl in the American diet. Overuse of salt can lead to serious medical conditions—including hardening of the arteries, heart attack, and stroke. Intake must be carefully monitored. In contrast, potassium is less abundantly supplied than its fellow electrolytes and can be dangerously depleted from body tissue through the use of diuretic medications—a condition that can prove permanently injurious or lethal. Being certain of obtaining adequate quantities of potassium while limiting your intake of sodium chloride is of considerable nutritional importance.

Estimated Safe and Adequate Daily Dietary Intakes of Selected Minerals[a]

| | Age (years) | Electrolytes | | |
		Sodium (mg)	Potassium (mg)	Chloride (mg)
Infants	0.0–0.5	115–350	350–925	275–700
	0.5–1.0	250–750	425–1275	400–1200
Children	1–3	325–975	550–1650	500–1500
and	4–6	450–1350	775–2325	700–2100
Adolescents	7–10	600–1800	1000–3000	925–2775
	11+	900–2700	1525–4575	1400–4200
Adults		1100–3300	1875–5625	1700–5100

From *Recommended Dietary Allowances,* Food and Nutrition Board, National Academy of Sciences-National Research Council, 1980.

[a] Because there is less information on which to base allowances, these figures are not given in the main table of RDA and are provided here in the form of ranges of recommended intakes.

A Selected List of Multivitamin Supplements

Key: Units: IU = international units; mg = milligrams; mcg = micrograms.
Vitamins: Vitamin D (calciferol, cholecalciferol, or ergocalciferol); Vitamin E (tocopherol); Vitamin B₁ (thiamin or thiamine); Vitamin B₂ (riboflavin); Vitamin B₃ (niacin, niacinamide, nicotinic acid, or nicotinamide); Vitamin B₆ (pyridoxine); Vitamin B₁₂ (cobalamin or cyanocobalamin); Pantothenic Acid (panthenol, calcium pantothenate, pantothenyl alcohol, or dexpanthenol).
Minerals: Ca (calcium); P (phosphorus); I (iodine); Fe (iron); Mg (magnesium); Zn (zinc); K (potassium); Mn (manganese).

Product (Manufacturer)	Vitamin A (IU)	Vitamin D (IU)	Vitamin E (IU)	Vitamin C (mg)	Folic Acid (mcg)	Vitamin B₁ (mg)	Vitamin B₂ (mg)	Vitamin B₃ (mg)	Vitamin B₆ (mg)	Vitamin B₁₂ (mcg)	Biotin (mcg)	Pantothenic Acid (mg)	Minerals & Other Nutrients[a] (mg unless noted)
A & D Halibut Liver Oil (Nu Life)	10,000	250	x	x	x	x	x	x	x	x	x	x	x
A to Zinc (Alacer)	3,333	67	33	250	133	6.7	6.7	10	6.7	67	33	13.3	Ca, 33; Cu, .17; I, .05; Fe, 6; Mg, 33; Zn, 1.7; K, 20; Mn, 66.7; Selenium, 6.7; Molybdenum, 66.7; Chromium, 6.7; Cho., 16.7; inos., 8.3; PABA, 6.7; leci., 16.7; nucleic acid, 23; yeast, 166.7

	A	D	E	C	FA	B$_1$	B$_2$	B$_3$	B$_6$	B$_{12}$	Bio	PA	Minerals/Other
AAA Herbal (Westpro)	x	x	x	100	x	x	x	100	x	x	x	x	x
Abdec (Parke-Davis)	10,000	400	5	75	x	5	3	25	1.5	2	x	10	
Abdec Baby Drops[b] (Parke-Davis)	5,000	400	x	50	x	1	1.2	10	1	x	x	5	x
Abdec Teens (Parke-Davis)	7,500	400	30	80	x	4.5	5.1	60	6	6	x	x	x
Abdol with Vitamin C (Parke-Davis)	5,000	400	x	50	x	2.5	2.5	20	.5	1	x	5	x
Action B-100 (Schein)	x	x	x	x	100	100	100	100	100	100	100	100	Cho., 100; inos., 100; PABA, 30
Adabee (Robins)	10,000	x	x	250	x	15	10	50	5	x	x	x	x
Adavite (Hudson)	10,000	400	15	187	x	10	10	100	5	5	x	18	x

For footnotes, see page 302.

A Selected List of Multivitamin Supplements (continued)

Product (Manufacturer)	Vitamin A (IU)	Vitamin D (IU)	Vitamin E (IU)	Vitamin C (mg)	Folic Acid (mcg)	Vitamin B1 (mg)	Vitamin B2 (mg)	Vitamin B3 (mg)	Vitamin B6 (mg)	Vitamin B12 (mcg)	Biotin (mcg)	Pantothenic Acid (mg)	Minerals & Other Nutrients[a] (mg unless noted)
A-Kare (Naturade)	8,333	x	10	30	x	x	20	x	3.3	x	x	x	Biof., 10; leci, 20
All 4 + 5 (Plus)	x	x	x	x	x	8.3	8.3	x	8.3	8.3	x	8.3	K, 8.3; Leci., 400; kelp, 25; vinegar, 50
All Natural Vitamin-A (Stur-Dee)	25,000	400	x	x	x	x	x	x	x	x	x	x	x
Allbee with C (Robins)	x	x	x	300	x	15	10	50	5	x	x	10	x
Allbee-T (Robins)	x	x	x	500	x	15	10	100	10	5	x	25	Liver, 150
Anorexin (SDA)	1,667	133	x	20	x	1	1	7	.3	.3	x	.3	Phenylpropanolamine, 25; caffeine, 100
Anti-Ox (Da Vinci)	1,000	40	100	250	x	x	x	x	x	x	x	x	Zn, 10; Selenium, .05; Chromium, .01; Meth., 50

	A	D	E	C	FA	B₁	B₂	B₃	B₆	B₁₂	Bio	PA	Minerals/Other
Anti-X (RichLife)	x	x	x	500	x	x	x	500	x	x	x	x	Glut. acid, 200
Ayds Multivits. & Mins. for Dieters (Campana)	5,000	400	30	90	400	12	10.2	25	12	200	15	25	Cu, 2; Fe, 18; Zn, 15; K 25
Aye-Aye (Westpro)	3,333	x	10	30	x	x	20	x	x	x	x	x	Biof., 5
B & C 800 (P. Leiner/Your Life)	x	x	45	800	x	15	17	100	25	12	x	25	x
B Complex (Plus)	x	x	x	x	16.7	.83	.83	8.3	.83	2.5	4.17	16.7	Cho., 166.7; inos., 166.7; PABA, 5
B Complex (Radiance)	x	x	x	x	133	2	2	16.7	.7	2	8.3	3.3	Cho., 16.7; inos., 16.7; PABA, 3
B Complex (Shaklee)	x	x	x	x	400	6.75	7.65	90	9	27	300	45	x
B Complex (Squibb)	x	x	x	x	x	.64	.66	8.1	.9	1	x	x	x

For footnotes, see page 302.

A Selected List of Multivitamin Supplements (continued)

Product (Manufacturer)	Vitamin A (IU)	Vitamin D (IU)	Vitamin E (IU)	Vitamin C (mg)	Folic Acid (mcg)	Vitamin B₁ (mg)	Vitamin B₂ (mg)	Vitamin B₃ (mg)	Vitamin B₆ (mg)	Vitamin B₁₂ (mcg)	Biotin (mcg)	Pantothenic Acid (mg)	Minerals & Other Nutrients[a] (mg unless noted)
B Complex Elixir (Schein)	x	x	x	x	x	7	3	20	1	x	x	x	x
B Complex w/C (Squibb)	x	x	x	300	x	10	10	100	2	4	x	x	x
B Complex w/C (Thompson)	x	x	x	150	200	5	5	50	5	37.5	15	25	Cho, 50; inos., 50; PABA, 15
B Complex w/ C 550 (Wampole)	x	x	x	550	x	25	12.5	60	10	x	x	10	x
B Compound w/ C Forte (Wampole)	x	x	x	300	x	35	15	50	5	10	x	20	x
Balanced B 50 Complex with C (RichLife)	x	x	x	50	100	50	50	50	50	50	50	50	Cho., 50; inos., 50; PABA, 50

250

	A	D	E	C	FA	B₁	B₂	B₃	B₆	B₁₂	Bio	PA	Minerals/Other
Balanced B-100 (Naturade)	x	x	x	x	400	100	100	100	100	100	100	100	Cho., 100; inos., 100; PABA, 100
Balanced B-100 Complex (Vita-Fresh)	x	x	x	x	100	100	100	100	100	100	100	100	x
Basic Vitalizer (Taylor)	.250	100	7.5	22	100	.52	.6	5	.5	2.25	75	2.5	Ca, 150; P, 70.5; Cu, 5; I, .04; Fe, 4.5; Mg, 50; Zn, 3.75; Mn, 1.75; Cho., 5; inos., 5; PABA, 3.75; biot., .75; leci., 5
Bayol (Vitamin Quota)	x	x	x	75	x	5	5	30	.5	3	x	2	Fe, 50
B-Calm (Vitamin Quota)	x	x	30	750	x	15	15	100	5	5	x	18.3	x
B-C-Bid (Geriatric)	x	x	x	300	x	5	10	50	5	5	x	10	x
B-Complex 50 (Plus)	x	x	x	x	100	50	50	50	50	50	50	50	Cho., 50; inos., 50; PABA, 30

For footnotes, see page 302.

A Selected List of Multivitamin Supplements (continued)

Product (Manufacturer)	Vitamin A (IU)	Vitamin D (IU)	Vitamin E (IU)	Vitamin C (mg)	Folic Acid (mcg)	Vitamin B$_1$ (mg)	Vitamin B$_2$ (mg)	Vitamin B$_3$ (mg)	Vitamin B$_6$ (mg)	Vitamin B$_{12}$ (mcg)	Biotin (mcg)	Pantothenic Acid (mg)	Minerals & Other Nutrients[a] (mg unless noted)
B-Complex 75 (Plus)	x	x	x	x	100	75	75	75	75	75	75	75	Cho., 75; inos., 75; PABA, 30
B-Complex 100 (Plus)	x	x	x	x	100	100	100	100	100	100	100	100	Cho., 100; inos., 100; PABA, 30
B-Complex Syrup with Iron (Plus)	x	x	x	x	100	5	5	30	5	10	15	50	Fe, 20; Cho., 60; inos., 60; PABA, 30
Becotin (Dista)	x	x	x	x-	x	10	10	50	4.1	1	x	25	x
Becotin with Vitamin C (Dista)	x	x	x	150	x	10	10	50	4.1	1	x	25	x
Becotin-T (Dista)	x	x	x	300	x	15	10	100	5	.4	x	20	x
Beminal-500 (Ayerst)	x	x	x	500	x	25	12.5	100	10	5	x	20	x

	A	D	E	C	FA	B_1	B_2	B_3	B_6	B_{12}	Bio	PA	Minerals/Other
Betalin (Lilly)	x	x	x	x	x	1	2	10	.4	1	x	3.33	x
Betalin Complex Elixir (Lilly)	x	x	x	x	x	2.7	1.35	6.75	.56	1.35	x	2.7	Liver, 540; alcohol, 17%
B-Folia (Naturade)	x	x	x	x	300	130	33	150	33	33	33	100	K, 33; Cho., 100; inos., 100; PABA, 33
B-Guard (Schiff)	x	x	x	x	x	7.5	10	15	6	.01	25	3	Cho., 1.71; inos., 1.95; PABA, .04
Big 100 Time Release (GNC/Nat. Sales)	x	x	x	x	400	100	100	100	100	100	100	100	Cho., 100; inos., 100; PABA, 30
Big 150 (GNC/Nat. Sales)	x	x	x	x	400	150	150	150	150	150	150	150	Cho., 150; inos., 150; PABA, 30
Brewer's Yeast (Prescription Labs.)	x	x	x	x	x	.18	.06	.6	x	x	x	x	x

For footnotes, see page 302.

A Selected List of Multivitamin Supplements (continued)

Product (Manufacturer)	Vitamin A (IU)	Vitamin D (IU)	Vitamin E (IU)	Vitamin C (mg)	Folic Acid (mcg)	Vitamin B$_1$ (mg)	Vitamin B$_2$ (mg)	Vitamin B$_3$ (mg)	Vitamin B$_6$ (mg)	Vitamin B$_{12}$ (mcg)	Biotin (mcg)	Pantothenic Acid (mg)	Minerals & Other Nutrients[a] (mg unless noted)
Brewer's Yeast Flakes[a] (Schiff)	x	x	x	x	90	4.28	1.14	11.4	1.14	2	25	1.42	Ca, 60; Fe, 2.5; K, 540; Cho, 100; inos, 100; PABA, .14
B-Stress with C (Solar)	x	x	x	250	100	5	5	50	5	12.5	12.5	50	Cho, 50; inos, 50; PABA, 15; brewer's yeast, 50
C & E-1000 (Basic Organics)	x	x	500	500	x	x	x	x	x	x	x	x	x
Cardenz (Miller)	2,000	100	5	25	x	x	x	20	1.5	1	x	x	I, .05; Mg, 23; K, 8; PABA, 9
C.E.B.-All (Schiff)	x	x	30	150	x	7	14	4.3	x	25	x	x	Biof., 35
Cebēfortis (Upjohn)	x	x	x	150	x	5	5	51	1	2	x	10	x
Cebētinic (Upjohn)	x	x	x	25	x	2	2	10	.5	5	x	x	Fe, 38

	A	D	E	C	FA	B₁	B₂	B₃	B₆	B₁₂	Bio	PA	Minerals/Other
Ceebevim (Hudson)	x	x	x	x	300	15	15	50	5	x	x	10	x
Centrum (Lederle)	5,000	400	30	90	400	2.25	2.6	20	3	9	150	10	Ca, 162; P, 125; Cu, 3; I, .15; Fe, 27; Mg, 100, Zn, 22.5; K, 7.5; Mn, 7.5
Century-B-100 (Basic Organics)	x	x	x	x	125	100	100	100	100	100	100	100	Cho., 100; inos., 100; PABA, 100
Chelated Iron Supreme (GNC)	x	x	x	30	x	1	x	.27	8.2	7	.5	.03	Fe, 25; Cho., 1; inos., 1.2; PABA, 6.8; biof., 15; liver, 31.2; lysine, .05
Cherry Cod Liver Oil[d] (Nu Life)	4,000	400	x	x	x	x	x	x	x	x	x	x	x
Chew-Vite (North American)	5,000	400	x	50	x	3	2.5	20	1	1	x	x	x
Child Love (Synergy Plus)	2,000	200	5	30	x	1.5	1.5	.86	1.5	5	x	1.5	Cu, .05; I, .015; Fe, 1; Mg, 3; Zn, .05; Mn, .2

For footnotes, see page 302.

255

A Selected List of Multivitamin Supplements (continued)

Product (Manufacturer)	Vitamin A (IU)	Vitamin D (IU)	Vitamin E (IU)	Vitamin C (mg)	Folic Acid (mcg)	Vitamin B₁ (mg)	Vitamin B₂ (mg)	Vitamin B₃ (mg)	Vitamin B₆ (mg)	Vitamin B₁₂ (mcg)	Biotin (mcg)	Pantothenic Acid (mg)	Minerals & Other Nutrients[a] (mg unless noted)
Children's Chewable Vits. (Nature's Bounty)	2,500	400	15	60	300	1.05	1.2	13.5	1.05	4.5	x	x	x
Children's Chewable Vits. w/Iron (Naturade)	5,000	400	15	75	10	4	4	10	4	10	50	10	Ca, 20; Cu, .07; I, .1; Fe, 5; Mg, .108; Zn, .05; Mn, .028; PABA, 4
Chocks & Chocks—Bugs Bunny (Miles)	2,500	400	15	60	300	1.05	1.2	13.5	1.05	4.5	x	x	x
Cluvisol & Cluvisol 130 (Ayerst)	10,000	400	.5	150	x	10	5	50	.5	2.5	x	1	Ca, 120; Fe, 15; Mg, 3; Zn, 6; Mn, .5
Cluvisol Syrup (Ayerst)	2,500	400	x	15	x	1	1	5	.6	2	x	3	Mg, 3; Zn, .5; Mn, .5

	A	D	E	C	FA	B₁	B₂	B₃	B₆	B₁₂	Bio	PA	Minerals/Other
Cod Liver Oil[a] (Squibb)	4,000	400	x	x	x	x	x	x	x	x	x	x	x
Cod Liver Oil, Mint-Flavored[d] (Squibb)	4,000	400	x	x	x	x	x	x	x	x	x	x	x
Cod Liver Oil Concentrate Capsules (Schering)	10,000	400	x	x	x	x	x	x	x	x	x	x	x
Combex (Parke-Davis)	x	x	x	x	x	10	10	10	x	1	x	6	Liver, 380
Combex with Vitamin C (Parke-Davis)	x	x	x	50	x	10	10	10	x	1	x	6	Liver, 340
Dayalets (Abbott)	5,000	400	30	60	400	1.5	1.7	20	2	6	x	x	
Delecta Yeast Flakes[f] (Schiff)	x	x	x	x	100	6	2	10	4	x	25	60	K, 200; Cho, 40; inos., 40; PABA, .13

For footnotes, see page 302.

A Selected List of Multivitamin Supplements (continued)

Product (Manufacturer)	Vitamin A (IU)	Vitamin D (IU)	Vitamin E (IU)	Vitamin C (mg)	Folic Acid (mcg)	Vitamin B_1 (mg)	Vitamin B_2 (mg)	Vitamin B_3 (mg)	Vitamin B_6 (mg)	Vitamin B_{12} (mcg)	Biotin (mcg)	Pantothenic Acid (mg)	Minerals & Other Nutrients[a] (mg unless noted)
De-Stress 21 (Vitamerica)	x	x	30	600	400	15	15	100	5	12	150	20	Fe, 7.5
Diastress (Radiance)	x	x	x	500	400	15	15	100	15	6	x	100	Biof., 60
Di*ET (Vita-Fresh)	5,000	400	15	60	400	1.5	1.7	20	2	6	150	10	Ca, 100; P, 100; Cu, 2; I, .15; Fe, 18; Mg, 100; Zn, 15; K, 10
Diet-Tab 21 (Vitamerica)	10,000	400	5	30	x	20	6	10	.5	10	1	3	Ca, 60; P, 45; Cu, 2; I, 1.11; Fe, 6; Mg, 1; Zn, 2; Mn, 3.4; Potassium chloride, 25; Liver, 100; yeast, 100
Double-Day (Schiff)	5,000	200	100	150	200	5	7.5	12.5	.05	12.5	325	.02	Ca, 187.5; P, 90; I, .04; Fe, 10; traces: Cu, Zn, Mn, Silicon, Fluorine; Cho., .85; inos., 1; PABA, .02; enzymes, 45
E.A.D.-All (Schiff)	5,000	400	75	x	x	x	x	x	x	x	x	x	x

	A	D	E	C	FA	B1	B2	B3	B6	B12	Bio	PA	Minerals/Other
Emergen-C (Alacer)	x	x	x	1,000	x	.38	.43	5	.5	1.5	x	2.5	Ca, 50; Mg, 20; Zn, 2; K, 125; Mn, 2; Selenium, .01; Sodium, 50
En-Cebrin Prenatal (Lilly)	4,000	400	x	50	x	3	2	10	1.7	5	x	5	Ca, 250; Cu, 1; I, .15; Fe, 30; Mg, 5; Zn, 1.5; Mn, 1
Energy 80 (Da Vinci/SportScience)	x	x	x	250	25	x	x	x	25	100	x	25	Mg, 50; Cho., 25; inos., 20; PABA, 25; leci., 150; betaine, 20; glut., 150; meth., 150; aspartic acid, 200
Engran-HP (Squibb)	4,000	200	15	30	x	.85	1	10	1.25	4	x	x	Ca, 325; I, .075; Fe, 9; Mg, 50
Essential B-Complex (RVP)	x	x	x	x	x	5	6	8	.4	x	x	.08	Cho., 2.7; inos., 3.43; PABA, .02
Exec-Power (Synergy Plus)	2,500	100	75	125	25	5	5	25	5	25	2.5	25	Fe, 2.5; Zn, 3.75; PABA, 5; leci., 125
Feminins (Mead Johnson)	5,000	400	10	200	100	1.5	3	15	25	10	x	10	Fe, 18; Zn, 10
Femiron with Vitamins (J. B. Williams)	5,000	400	x	60	100	1.5	1.7	20	2	5	x	10	Fe, 20

For footnotes, see page 302.

A Selected List of Multivitamin Supplements (continued)

Product (Manufacturer)	Vita-min A (IU)	Vita-min D (IU)	Vita-min E (IU)	Vita-min C (mg)	Folic Acid – (mcg)	Vita-min B1 (mg)	Vita-min B2 (mg)	Vita-min B3 (mg)	Vita-min B6 (mg)	Vita-min B12 (mcg)	Bio-tin – (mcg)	Panto-thenic Acid – (mg)	Minerals & Other Nutrients[a] (mg unless noted)
Filibon Capsules (Lederle)	5,000	400	30	60	400	1.5	1.7	20	2	6	x	x	Ca, 125; I, 15; Fe, 18; Mg, 100
Filibon F. A. (Lederle)	8,000	400	30	60	800	1.7	2	20	4	8	x	x	Ca, 250; I, 15; Fe, 45; Mg, 100; DSS, 100
Flavored Yeast (Squibb)	x	x	x	x	x	.9	.34	3	x	x	x	x	Protein, 2% RDA
Flintstones (Miles)	2,500	400	15	60	300	1.05	1.2	13.5	1.05	4.5	x	x	x
Flintstones plus Iron (Miles)	2,500	400	15	60	300	1.05	1.2	13.5	1.05	4.5	x	x	Fe, 15
Folic Acid and B12 (Plus)	x	x	x	x	100 400	x	x	x	x	1 40	x	x	x
Formula B-Complex "50" (Solgar)	x	x	x	x	100	50	50	50	50	50	50	50	Cho., 50; inos., 50; PABA, 50

	A	D	E	C	FA	B_1	B_2	B_3	B_6	B_{12}	Bio	PA	Minerals/Other
Fortespan (Smith Kline & French)	10,000	400	x	150	x	6	6	60	6	15	x	x	x
Fumatinic (Laser)	x	x	30	200	100	10	10	20	3	15	x	10	Fe, 100
Ganatrex[b] (Merrell-National)	5,000	400	30	60	x	1.5	1.7	20	2	6	x	x	Alcohol, 15%; invert sugar
Gems (Naturite)	5,000	400	15	60	400	1.5	1.7	20	2	6	x	x	Fe, 18
Geriban (Hudson)	x	x	x	75	x	5	5	30	.5	3	x	2	Fe, 2
Geribom (Bowman)	10,000	400	2	75	x	5	2.5	40	1	2	x	4	Ca, 75; P, 58; Fe, 30; Mg, 3; Zn, .5; K, 2; Mn, 3; Cho., 31.4; inos., 15
Gerilets (Abbott)	5,000	400	45	90	400	2.25	2.6	30	3	9	450	15	Fe, 27

For footnotes, see page 302.

A Selected List of Multivitamin Supplements (continued)

Product (Manufacturer)	Vitamin A (IU)	Vitamin D (IU)	Vitamin E (IU)	Vitamin C (mg)	Folic Acid — (mcg)	Vitamin B1 (mg)	Vitamin B2 (mg)	Vitamin B3 (mg)	Vitamin B6 (mg)	Vitamin B12 (mcg)	Biotin — (mcg)	Pantothenic Acid — (mg)	Minerals & Other Nutrients[a] (mg unless noted)
Gerimost (Schiff)	1,667	67	17	33	x	1.17	2.33	.75	.01	4.17	x	.02	Ca, 91.7; P, 66.7; I, .01; Fe, 6.7; Mg, 6.7; traces: Zn, Silicon; Cho., .58; inos., .7; biof., 6.7; nucleic acid, 15; glut., 15; enzymes, 26
Geriplex (Parke-Davis)	5,000	x	5	50	x	5	5	15	x	2	x	x	Ca, 59; P, 46; Cu, 4; Fe, 6; Zn, 2; Mn, 4; Cho., 20; enzymes, 162.5
Geriplex-FS (Parke-Davis)	5,000	x	5	50	x	5	5	15	x	2	x	x	Ca, 59; P, 46; Cu, 4; Fe, 6; Zn, 2; Mn, 4; Cho., 20; enzymes, 162.5; DSS, 100
Geriplex-FS Liquid† (Parke-Davis)	x	x	x	x	x	1.2	1.7	15	1	5	x	x	Fe, 15; Fecal softeners, 200; alcohol, 18%
Geritol Liquid† (J. B. Williams)	x	x	x	x	x	5	5	100	1	3	x	4	Fe, 100; Cho., 41.18; meth., 75
Geritol Tablets (J. B. Williams)	x	x	x	75	x	5	5	30	.5	3	x	2	Fe, 50

	A	D	E	C	FA	B₁	B₂	B₃	B₆	B₁₂	Bio	PA	Minerals/Other
Gerix Elixir† (Abbott)	x	x	x	x	x	6	6	200	2	6	x	x	Fe, 15; Cho., 200; inos., 200; betaine, 100
Gevrabon† (Lederle)	x	x	x	x	x	5	2.5	50	1	1	x	10	I, 1; Fe, 20; Mg, 2; Zn, 2; Mn, 2; Cho., 100; inos., 100; alcohol, 18%
Gevral (Lederle)	5,000	400	30	60	400	1.5	1.7	20	2	6	x	5	Ca, 162; P, 125; I, .15; Fe, 18; Mg, 100
Gevral T (Lederle)	5,000	400	45	90	400	2.25	2.6	30	3	9	x	x	Ca, 162; P, 125; Cu, 1.5; I, .225; Fe, 27; Mg, 100; Zn, 22.5
Gevrite (Lederle)	5,000	x	x	60	x	1.5	1.7	20	2	x	x	x	Ca, 230; Fe, 18
Golden Bounty B Complex with Vita. C (Squibb)	x	x	x	100	x	4	4.8	4.67	x	25	x	x	x
Golden Bounty Brewer's Yeast Tablets (Squibb)	x	x	x	x	x	.18	.06	.6	x	x	x	x	x
Golden Bounty Multivitamin Supplement w/Iron (Squibb)	5,000	400	30	60	400	1.5	1.7	20	2	6	x	x	Fe, 18

For footnotes, see page 302.

A Selected List of Multivitamin Supplements (continued)

Product (Manufacturer)	Vitamin A (IU)	Vitamin D (IU)	Vitamin E (IU)	Vitamin C (mg)	Folic Acid (mcg)	Vitamin B₁ (mg)	Vitamin B₂ (mg)	Vitamin B₃ (mg)	Vitamin B₆ (mg)	Vitamin B₁₂ (mcg)	Biotin (mcg)	Pantothenic Acid (mg)	Minerals & Other Nutrients[a] (mg unless noted)
Halibut Liver Oil (Schiff)	5,000	85	x	x	x	x	x	x	x	x	x	x	x
Hemotinic Iron Formula (RichLife)	x	x	x	100	33	5	5	30	5	16.7	x	1.8	Cu, .28; Fe, 40; Mn, .11; Liver, 454
Hep-Forte (Marlyn)	1,200	x	10	10	60	1	1	10	.5	1	3.3	2	Zn, 2; Cho, 10; inos., 10; meth., 10; yeast, 64.8; liver, 328
Hepicebrin (Lilly)	5,000	400	x	75	x	2	3	20	x	x	x	x	x
Hi B (Westpro)	x	x	x	x	50	50	25	50	25	25	25	50	Cho, 50; inos., 50; PABA, 15; yeast, 50; liver, 50
Hi-B-Com (Richards)	x	x	x	x	x	7	14	4	x	10	x	x	x
Hi-B-Complex Tablets & Capsules (Schiff)	x	x	x	x	2	3	6	1	.02	5	.5	.04	Cho, 1.7; inos., 2; PABA, .01

	A	D	E	C	FA	B_1	B_2	B_3	B_6	B_{12}	Bio	PA	Minerals/Other
Hi-B-Complex 100 (Hudson)	x	x	x	x	400	100	100	100	100	100	100	100	x
Hi Po A & D (Thompson)	25,000	1,000		x	x	x	x	x	x	x	x	x	x
High Potency Liver, Iron and B-12 (Hall's)	x	x	x	75	50	x	x	x	x	15	x	x	Fe, 50; Liver, 400
High-Potency B-Complex and C (Plus)	x	x	x	150	50	5	5	50	5	12.5	12.5	25	Cho., 50; inos., 50; PABA, 30
High-Potency B-Complex with C (Plus)	x	x	x	500	50	10	10	20	10	5	10	100	PABA, 10
Hi-Potency B-Complex w/Vit. C (Naturite)	x	x	x	150	200	5	5	50	5	37.5	15	25	Cho., 50; inos., 5; PABA, 15
High Potency Vitalizer (Taylor)	2,500	133	20	100	133	5	5	16.7	5	10	100	16.7	Ca, 200; P, 94; Cu, 67; I, .05; Fe, 6; Mg, 66.7; Zn, 3; Mn, 2.3; Cho., 16.7; inos., 16.7; PABA, 10; biot., 2; leci, 13.3

For footnotes, see page 302.

A Selected List of Multivitamin Supplements (continued)

Product (Manufacturer)	Vitamin A (IU)	Vitamin D (IU)	Vitamin E (IU)	Vitamin C (mg)	Folic Acid (mcg)	Vitamin B1 (mg)	Vitamin B2 (mg)	Vitamin B3 (mg)	Vitamin B6 (mg)	Vitamin B12 (mcg)	Biotin (mcg)	Pantothenic Acid (mg)	Minerals & Other Nutrients[a] (mg unless noted)
Hi-Yeast (Biorganic)	x	x	x	x	x	3	6	1	.02	10	.5	trace	P, 6; Mg, 1.8; K, 7; Cho, 1.5; inos., .2
Homicebrin[d] (Lilly)	3,000	400	x	60	x	1	1.2	10	.8	3	x	x	Alcohol, 5%
Hyalex (Miller)	1,500	350	3	30	x	x	x	x	x	2	x	5	Mg, 5; Zn, .7
Hypo-Plex (Nature's Plus)	2,500	x	x	500	x	25	25	x	25	25	x	100	x
Iberet (Abbott)	x	x	x	150	x	6	6	30	5	25	x	10	Fe, 105
Iberet Liquid[d] (Abbott)	x	x	x	37.5	x	1.5	1.5	7.5	1.25	6.25	x	2.5	Fe, 26.25
Iberet-500 (Abbott)	x	x	x	500	x	6	6	30	5	25	x	10	Fe, 105
Iberet-500 Liquid[d] (Abbott)	x	x	x	125	x	1.5	1.5	7.5	1.25	6.25	x	2.5	Fe, 26.25
Iberol (Abbott)	x	x	x	75	x	3	3	15	1.5	12.5	x	3	Fe, 105

266

	A	D	E	C	FA	B₁	B₂	B₃	B₆	B₁₂	Bio	PA	Minerals/Other
Iberol-F (Abbott)	x	x	x	75	200	3	3	15	1.5	12.5	x	3	Fe, 105
Initia Drops[b] (Parke-Davis)	1,500	200	x	x	50	x	x	x	1	x	x	x	x
Junior-Vite (Basic Organics)	2,000	200	5	x	30	1.6	1.5	.9	1.6	5	x	1.6	Cu, .05; I, .015; Fe, 1.05; Mg, .31; Zn, .06; Mn, 21
Lactocal (Laser)	5,000	400	x	60	800	3	2	20	10	8	x	10	Ca, 160; Cu, 2; Fe, 33; Mg, 10; Zn, 15
Lederplex Capsules (Lederle)	x	x	x	x	x	2.25	2.6	30	3	9	x	15	x
Lederplex Liquid[d] (Lederle)	x	x	x	x	x	1.13	1.3	15	1.5	4.5	x	7.5	x
Lederplex Tablets (Lederle)	x	x	x	x	x	2	2	10	.1	1	x	3	x
Liqui-Lea[d] (Shaklee)	5,000	400	15	x	x	2.1	1.8	20	2	9	300	5	Fe, 18

For footnotes, see page 302.

267

A Selected List of Multivitamin Supplements (continued)

Product (Manufacturer)	Vitamin A (IU)	Vitamin D (IU)	Vitamin E (IU)	Vitamin C (mg)	Folic Acid (mcg)	Vitamin B₁ (mg)	Vitamin B₂ (mg)	Vitamin B₃ (mg)	Vitamin B₆ (mg)	Vitamin B₁₂ (mcg)	Biotin (mcg)	Pantothenic Acid (mg)	Minerals & Other Nutrients[a] (mg unless noted)
Lipoflavonoid (Smith, Miller & Patch)	x	x	x	100	x	.3	.3	3.3	.3	1.7	x	.3	Cho, 233; biof., 100
Lipotriad Liquid (Smith, Miller & Patch)	x	x	x	x	x	1	1	10	1	.5	x	1	x
Livitamin Capsules (Beecham)	x	x	x	100	x	3	3	10	3	5	x	2	Cu, .66; Fe, 33; Liver, 150
Livitamin Chewable Tabs. (Beecham)	x	x	x	100	x	3	3	10	3	5	x	2	Cu, .33; Fe, 16.4
Livitamin Liquide (Beecham)	x	x	x	x	x	3	3	10	3	5	x	2	Cu, .66; Fe, 35.5; Liver, 500

	A	D	E	C	FA	B₁	B₂	B₃	B₆	B₁₂	Bio	PA	Minerals/Other
Livitamin Prenatal Tablets (Beecham)	6,000	400	x	100	500	3	3	20	10	5	x	5	Ca, 350; Fe, 50
Magna B B-Complex 100 (Radiance)	x	x	x	x	400	100	100	100	100	100	100	100	Cho., 100; inos., 10; PABA, 100
Maxim-All/ Maxim-All PRN (Am. Dietaids)	25,000	1,000	150	300	400	80	80	80	80	80	80	80	Ca, 50; Cu, .25; I, .15; Fe, 10; Mg, 7.2; Zn, 15; K, 10; Mn, 6.1; Cho., 80; inos., 40; PABA, 80; biot., 55; glut. acid, 25; betaine, 25; chlorophyll, 2
Mega B-75 (Nature's Plus)	x	x	x	x	100	75	75	75	75	75	75	75	Cho., 75; inos., 75; PABA, 30
Mega Formula B Complex 75 (RichLife)	x	x	x	x	100	75	75	75	75	75	75	75	Cho., 75; inos., 75; PABA, 75
Mega Caps (P. Leiner/Your Life)	10,000	400	60	150	200	25	25	25	20	25	25	25	Ca, 100; P, 25; Cu, 1; I, .075; Fe, 9; Mg, 25; Zn, 3; K, 3; Mn, 1; Selenium, .005; Cho., 10; inos., 10; PABA, 10; leci., 10

For footnotes, see page 302.

A Selected List of Multivitamin Supplements (continued)

Product (Manufacturer)	Vita-min A (IU)	Vita-min D (IU)	Vita-min E (IU)	Vita-min C (mg)	Folic Acid (mcg)	Vita-min B1 (mg)	Vita-min B2 (mg)	Vita-min B3 (mg)	Vita-min B6 (mg)	Vita-min B12 (mcg)	Bio-tin (mcg)	Panto-thenic Acid (mg)	Minerals & Other Nutrients[a] (mg unless noted)
Mega-One (GNC/Nat. Sales)	25,000	400	150	250	400	50	50	100	50	50	300	100	Ca, 10; Cu, 25; I, .15; Fe, 1; Mg, 54; Zn, 1.15; K, 1; Mn, 61; Cho., 250; inos., 250; PABA, 50; biof., 55; be-taine, 25; glut. acid, 25
Mega Plus (Westpro)	4,167	167	67	200	67	10	10	10	10	17	17	20	Ca, 166.7; P, 25; Cu, .33; I, .04; Fe, 3; Mg, 66.7; Zn, 3; K, 16.5; Mn, 3; Chromium, .03; Selenium, 25; Cho., 10; inos., 10; PABA, 10; biof., 10; betaine, 15; gland tissues, 30
Mega Stress Vites (Synergy Plus)	x			250	x	x	x	250	25	x	x	x	Glut, 100
Mega-V & M (Nature's Bounty)	25,000	1,000	100	250	400	80	80	80	80	80	80	80	Ca, 50; Cu, .5; I, .15; Fe, 10; Mg, 7; Zn, 25; K, 10; Mn, 6; Cho., 80; inos., 80; PABA, 80; biof., 65; betaine, 30; glut. acid, 30

	A	D	E	C	FA	B1	B2	B3	B6	B12	Bio	PA	Minerals/Other
Mega Vits. & Mins. (Vita-Fresh)	5,000	200	100	300	200	25	25	25	25	50	12.5	12.5	Ca, 75; P, 34; Cu, .05; I, .04; Fe, 9; Mg, 25; Zn, 15; K, 2.5; Mn, 2.5
Mevanin-C (Beutlich)	3,000	300	x	200	100	2	2	5	.5	1	x	x	Ca, 55; Cu, 34; I, 03; Fe, 14; Mg, 1; Zn, 42; K, 1.5; Mn, 35; Biof., 30
Mevatinic-C (Beutlich)	x	x	x	225	100	x	x	x	x	5	x	x	Cu, .33; Fe, 67; Zn, 4; Biof., 30
Mi-Cebrin (Dista)	10,000	400	5.5	100	x	10	5	30	1.7	3	x	10	Cu, 1; I, .15; Fe, 15; Mg, 5; Zn, 1.5; Mn, 1
Mi-Cebrin T (Dista)	10,000	400	5.5	150	x	15	10	100	2	7.5	x	10	Cu, 1; I, .15; Fe, 15; Mg, 5; Zn, 1.5; Mn, 1
Mission Prenatal F.A. (Mission)	4,000	400	x	100	800	5	2	10	10	2	x	1	Ca, 50; Fe, 38.6
Monster (Bristol-Myers)	3,500	400	x	40	100	1.1	1.2	15	1.2	5	x	5	x
Ms. Power (Synergy Plus)	2,500	200	15	100	50	.75	.9	10	25	12.5	x	25	Ca, 50; Fe, 9; Mg, 30; Zn, 7.5

For footnotes, see page 302.

271

A Selected List of Multivitamin Supplements (continued)

Product (Manufacturer)	Vita-min A (IU)	Vita-min D (IU)	Vita-min E (IU)	Vita-min C (mg)	Folic Acid — (mcg)	Vita-min B₁ (mg)	Vita-min B₂ (mg)	Vita-min B₃ (mg)	Vita-min B₆ (mg)	Vita-min B₁₂ (mcg)	Bio-tin — (mcg)	Panto-thenic Acid — (mg)	Minerals & Other Nutrients[a] (mg unless noted)
Mucoplex (Stuart)	x	x	x	x	x	x	1.5	x	x	5	x	x	Liver, 750
Muta-Gen 12+E (Bowman)	5,000	400	15	37	200	2	2	20	1	3	x	x	x
Multicebrin (Lilly)	10,000	400	6.6	75	x	3	3	25	1.2	3	x	5	x
Multivitamin Supplement w/Iron (Fisons)	5,000	x	30	60	400	1.5	1.7	20	2	6	x	x	Fe, 18
Multi-vitamins (Thompson)	4,000	400	x	75	x	1	1.2	10	2	2	x	x	Honey
Multivitamins plus Iron (Wampole)	5,000	400	x	50	x	2	3	20	1	3	x	x	Fe, 4
Multivitamins Rowell (Rowell)	5,000	400	10	50	x	2.5	2.5	20	.5	2	x	5	x

	A	D	E	C	FA	B₁	B₂	B₃	B₆	B₁₂	Bio	PA	Minerals/Other
Multohab (Bowman)	5,000	400	x	50	x	3	3	20	.5	1	x	5	x
Mulvidren (Stuart)	4,000	400	x	75	x	2	2	10	1.2	3	x	3	x
Mulvitab (Reid-Provident)	8,000	400	2	75	x	3	3	20	1	2	x	5	x
Myadec Capsules and Tablets (Parke-Davis)	10,000	400	30	250	x	10	10	100	5	5	x	x	Cu, 2; I, .15; Fe, 20; Mg, 25; Zn, 1.5, Mn, 1
Natabec-F.A. (Parke-Davis)	4,000	400	x	50	100	.3	2	10	3	5	x	x	Ca, 600; Fe, 55
Natalins (Mead Johnson)	8,000	400	30	90	800	1.7	2	20	4	8	x	x	Ca, 200; I, .15; Fe, 45; Mg, 100
Neofol B12 (Nion)	x	x	x	x	400	x	x	x	x	40	x	x	Brewer's yeast
Niarb-Super (Miller)	x	x	x	300	x	x	x	200	x	x	x	x	Mg, 50

For footnotes, see page 302.

A Selected List of Multivitamin Supplements (continued)

Product (Manufacturer)	Vitamin A (IU)	Vitamin D (IU)	Vitamin E (IU)	Vitamin C (mg)	Folic Acid (mcg)	Vitamin B$_1$ (mg)	Vitamin B$_2$ (mg)	Vitamin B$_3$ (mg)	Vitamin B$_6$ (mg)	Vitamin B$_{12}$ (mcg)	Biotin (mcg)	Pantothenic Acid (mg)	Minerals & Other Nutrients[a] (mg unless noted)
Norlac (Rowell)	8,000	400	30	90	400	2	2	20	4	8	x	x	Ca, 200; Cu, 2; I, .15; Fe, 60; Mg, 100; Zn, 15
Novacebrin Chewable (Lilly)	4,000	400	x	60	x	1.5	2	12	.8	3	x	2.5	x
Novacebrin Drops[b] (Lilly)	4,000	400	x	60	x	1	1	10	.8	x	x	x	x
Nucle-B.E.C. (Schiff)	x	x	50	100	x	5	10	3	x	2.5	x	x	RNA, 100
Nuclomin (Miller)	2,500	200	12.5	25	x	1.13	1.25	12.5	1.5	3	x	7.5	Cu, .5; I, .038; Fe, 5; Mg, 50; Zn, 3.75; Mn, 1.5
Nutri-B Complex (Nature Food Ctrs.)	x	x	x	x	400	10	15	25	10	25	100	100	Cho, 250; inos, 250; PABA, 50

274

	A	D	E	C	FA	B₁	B₂	B₃	B₆	B₁₂	Bio	PA	Minerals/Other
Nutri-Hair (Am. Dietaids)	x	x	5	x	x	x	x	35	x	6	105	100	Cu, 1; I, .15; Fe, 10; Zn, 15; Mn, 5; trace Chromium; Cho, 250; inos., 50; PABA, 30
Nutri-Mega (Radiance)	5,000	200	150	150	200	25	25	25	25	25	25	25	Ca, 100; P, .25; Cu, 1; I, .075; Fe, 9; Mg, 25; Zn, 7.5; K, 15; Mn, 15; Cho., 25; inos., 25; PABA, 25; leci., 40
Nuplex (Thompson)	10,000	400	30	200	400	10	10	100	10	15	x	20	Ca, 125; P, 96; Cu, 1; I, .15; Fe, 15; Mg, 8; Zn, 1.5; Mn, 1
Obron-6 (Pfipharmecs)	5,000	400	x	50	x	3.09	2	20.16	8.23	2	x	.92	Ca, 245; Fe, 35; Mg, 15; Zn, 4; K, 1.7; Mn, .33
Omni/Omni 2000 (Da Vinci/ SportScience)	5,000	66	133	333	100	20	20	20	20	5	66.7	20	Ca, 33; P, 16.7; Cu, 16.7; I, .01; Fe, 3.3; Mg, 33.3; Zn, 5; K, 16.7; Mn, 1.7; Selenium, 10; Chromium, 10; Molybdenum, 10; Cho., 20; inos., 20; PABA, 20; biot., 140; leci., 66.7; RNA, 20; pectin, 16.7
One A Meal (RichLife)	3,333	133	17	50	33	8.3	8.3	40	8.3	8.3	16.7	40	Ca, 67; P, 30; Cu, 17; I, .05; Fe, 7; Mg, 33; Zn, 2; K, 8.3; Mn, 2; Cho., 80; inos., 80; PABA, 10; biot., 58; betaine, 8.3; glut. acid, 20; lysine, 20; enzymes, 11.7

For footnotes, see page 302.

A Selected List of Multivitamin Supplements (continued)

Product (Manufacturer)	Vita-min A (IU)	Vita-min D (IU)	Vita-min E (IU)	Vita-min C (mg)	Folic Acid – (mcg)	Vita-min B₁ (mg)	Vita-min B₂ (mg)	Vita-min B₃ (mg)	Vita-min B₆ (mg)	Vita-min B₁₂ (mcg)	Bio-tin – (mcg)	Panto-thenic Acid – (mg)	Minerals & Other Nutrients[a] (mg unless noted)
One-A-Day (Miles)	5,000	400	15	60	400	1.5	1.7	20	2	6	x	x	x
One-A-Day plus Iron (Miles)	5,000	400	15	60	400	1.5	1.7	20	2	6	x	x	Fe, 18
One-A-Day plus Minerals (Miles)	5,000	400	15	60	400	1.5	1.7	20	2	6	x	10	Ca, 100; P, 100; Cu, 2; I, .15; Fe, 18; Mg, 100; Zn, 15
One-Up (Plus)	10,000	400	100	250	400	10	10	25	10	10	25	25	Ca, 80; P, 62; Cu, 5; I, 1; Fe, 13.5; Mg, 40; Zn, 4
On-the-Go (Origin)	5,000	400	30	90	400	5	5	40	4	12	x	20	Ca, 125; Cu, 2; I, .15; Fe, 50; Zn, 15; K, 7.5; Mn, 7.5
Optilets-500 (Abbott)	10,000	400	30	500	x	15	10	100	5	12	x	20	x
Ora-Scorbs (Alacer)	x	x	x	500	x	.75	.85	5	1	3	15	5	Selenium, 2; Chromium, 2; Glut., 40; lysine, 20

	A	D	E	C	FA	B₁	B₂	B₃	B₆	B₁₂	Bio	PA	Minerals/Other
Os-Cal Plus (Marion)	1,666	125	x	33	x	.5	.66	3.3	.5	.03	x	.3	Ca, 250; Cu, .036; I, 1.036; Fe, 16.6; Zn, .75; Mn, .75
Paladac Liquid[d] (Parke-Davis)	5,000	400	x	50	x	3	3	20	1	5	x	5	x
Paladac with Minerals (Parke-Davis)	4,000	400	10	50	x	3	3	20	1	5	x	5	Ca, 23; P, 17; I, .05; Fe, 5; Mg, 1; K, 2.5
Pals (Bristol-Myers)	3,500	400	x	60	50	.8	1.3	14	1	2.5	x	5	x
Peach Flavored Cod Liver Oil[h] (Superl)	3,750	380	x	x	x	x	x	x	x	x	x	x	x
Phospho Tonic[j] (Wampole)	x	x	x	x	x	.75	1.25	7.5	.35	x	x	x	
Polysorbin Chewable (Reid-Provident)	3,500	400	4	75	100	1.1	1.2	15	1.2	5	x	7	x

For footnotes, see page 302.

277

A Selected List of Multivitamin Supplements (continued)

Product (Manufacturer)	Vitamin A (IU)	Vitamin D (IU)	Vitamin E (IU)	Vitamin C (mg)	Folic Acid — (mcg)	Vitamin B₁ (mg)	Vitamin B₂ (mg)	Vitamin B₃ (mg)	Vitamin B₆ (mg)	Vitamin B₁₂ (mcg)	Biotin (mcg)	Pantothenic Acid — (mg)	Minerals & Other Nutrients[a] (mg unless noted)
Polysorbin Drops (Reid-Provident)	3,000	400	5	60	x	1	1.2	8	1	x	x	3	x
Poly-Vi-Sol (Mead Johnson)	2,500	400	15	60	300	1.05	1.2	13.5	1.05	4.5	x	x	x
Poly-Vi-Sol Drops (Mead Johnson)	1,500	400	5	35	x	.5	.6	8	.4	2	x	x	x
Poly-Vi-Sol with Iron (Mead Johnson)	2,500	400	15	60	300	1.05	1.2	13.5	1.05	4.5	x	x	Fe, 12
Poly-Vi-Sol with Iron Drops (Mead Johnson)	1,500	400	5	35	x	.5	.6	8	.4	x	x	x	Fe, 10
Pregent (Beutlich)	x	300	x	100	100	x	x	x	x	x	x	x	Ca, 120; Fe, 41; Biof., 10

	A	D	E	C	FA	B₁	B₂	B₃	B₆	B₁₂	Bio	PA	Minerals/Other
PreNatal (Westpro)	2,500	100	50	125	200	3.75	3.75	25	12.5	25	75	6.25	Ca, 187.5; P, 50; Cu, .5; I, .06; Fe, 5; Mg, 75; Zn, 3.75; K, 24.75; Mn, 2.5; Chromium, .05; Cho, 6.25; inos, 6.25; PABA, 7.5
Pre-teen Plex (Thompson)	3,750	200	22.5	45	200	1.1	1.3	15	1.5	4.5	22.5	7.5	Ca, 150; P, 75; I, .75; Fe, 5; Mg, 75; Zn, 5; Mn, 1.5; Cho, 25; inos, 25
Probec (Stuart)	x	x	x	250	x	15	10	50	5	3	x	10	x
Probec-T (Stuart)	x	x	x	600	x	15	10	100	5	5	x	20	x
Pro-Hair 21 (Vitamerica)	x	x	x	x	400	x	x	35	x	6	x	100	Cu, 2; I, .15; Fe, 9; Zn, 15; Mn, 1; Cho, 125; inos, 125; PABA, 30
Pure-Vite (Nature-Made)	5,000	400	x	60	x	2	2.1	8.4	.4	5	x	1.7	I, .017; Fe, 5; traces: Cu, Mg, Zn, K, Mn
Ragus (Miller)	1,667	133	3.3	33.3	x	6.7	1	26.6	1.7	3	x	1.7	Ca, 193; P, 150; Cu, .3; I, .033; Fe, 6.7; Mg, 9; Zn, .7; K, 3.3; Mn, .7; Lysine, 8.3; meth, 16.7
Ray-D (Nion)	x	67	x	x	x	.17	.33	1.7	x	x	x	x	Ca, 62.5; P, 50; I, .017; Brewer's yeast

For footnotes, see page 302.

A Selected List of Multivitamin Supplements (continued)

Product (Manufacturer)	Vita-min A (IU)	Vita-min D (IU)	Vita-min E (IU)	Vita-min C (mg)	Folic Acid – (mcg)	Vita-min B₁ (mg)	Vita-min B₂ (mg)	Vita-min B₃ (mg)	Vita-min B₆ (mg)	Vita-min B₁₂ (mcg)	Bio-tin – (mcg)	Panto-thenic Acid – (mg)	Minerals & Other Nutrients[a] (mg unless noted)
RDA Vit. Formula w/Mins. (Am. Dietaids)	5,000	400	30	60	400	1.5	1.7	20	2	6	x	10	Ca, 100; P, 100; Cu, 2; I, .15; Fe, 18; Mg, 100; Zn, 15
RoeriBeC (Pfipharmecs)	x	x	x	500	x	10	10	100	10	4	x	20	x
Sclerex (Miller)	833	67	2	33.3	33.3	1.7	.7	11.6	1.3	1	x	2.5	Ca, 8.3; Cu, .3; I, .033; Fe, 3.3; Mg, 8.8; Zn, 1; Mn, 3; Inos. 667
Scott's Emulsion[d] (Beecham)	1,000	100	x	x	x	x	x	x	x	x	x	x	Cod liver oil
Second Wind (Alacer)	1,000	25	20	100	20	5	5	5	5	20	20	5	Zn, 1; K, 150; Selenium, .01; Chromium, .002; Cho., 4; inos., 4; PABA, .004; leci, 10; amino acids, 10; kelp, 6; pectin, 5; yeast, 110; liver, 400
Sigtab (Upjohn)	5,000	400	15	333	33	10	10	100	2	4	x	20	x

	A	D	E	C	FA	B_1	B_2	B_3	B_6	B_{12}	Bio	PA	Minerals/Other
Skin (Natural Organics)	2,000	200	50	x	x	x	x	30	10	x	25	x	Zn, 1; PABA, 50
Smiles (Wampole)	5,000	400	x	50	x	2	x	x	1	3	x	x	x
Space Invaders (P. Leiner/Your Life)	2,500	400	15	250	300	1.05	1.2	13.5	1.05	4.5	x	x	x
Special Formula B-Complex 50 w/C (Radiance)	x	x	x	50	400	50	50	50	50	50	50	50	Cho., 50; inos., 10; PABA, 50
Spider-man (Hudson)	2,500	400	15	60	300	1.05	1.2	13.5	1.05	4.5	x	x	x
S.S.S. Tablets (S.S.S.)	x	x	x	75	x	5	2.4	30	.5	1.5	x	2	Cu, 1; Fe, 50
S.S.S. Tonic[c] (S.S.S.)	x	x	x	x	x	1.7	.8	6.7	x	x	x	x	Fe, 33.3; Alcohol, 12%
Strawberry Shortcake (Vita-Fresh)	2,500	400	15	60	300	1.05	1.2	13.5	1.05	4.5	x	x	x

For footnotes, see page 302.

281

A Selected List of Multivitamin Supplements (continued)

Product (Manufacturer)	Vita-min A (IU)	Vita-min D (IU)	Vita-min E (IU)	Vita-min C (mg)	Folic Acid — (mcg)	Vita-min B₁ (mg)	Vita-min B₂ (mg)	Vita-min B₃ (mg)	Vita-min B₆ (mg)	Vita-min B₁₂ (mcg)	Bio-tin — (mcg)	Panto-thenic Acid — (mg)	Minerals & Other Nutrients[a] (mg unless noted)
Stress B (Da Vinci/FoodScience)	x	x	x	x	x	55	55	55	55	9	x	15	x
Stress B (Da Vinci/SportScience)	x	x	x	x	200	55	55	200	55	12	100	55	Cho, 55; inos., 55; PABA, 55
Stress Formula (Wampole)	x	x	x	500	x	35	15	50	5	10	x	20	Fe, 10
Stress Formula & Zinc (P. Leiner/Your Life)	x	x	45	600	400	20	10	100	10	25	x	25	Cu, 3; Zn, 23.9
Stress Formula Caps. (Origin)	x	x	x	500	400	15	15	100	15	6	x	100	Biof., 60
Stress Formula 600 (Hudson)	x	x	30	600	x	15	15	100	5	12	x	20	x

	A	D	E	C	FA	B_1	B_2	B_3	B_6	B_{12}	Bio	PA	Minerals/Other
Stress Formula 600 with Iron (Genovese)	x	x	30	600	400	15	15	100	25	12	x	20	Fe, 27
Stress Formula 26 (RichLife)	x	x	x	250	50	5	5	50	5	12.5	12.5	50	Cho., 50; inos., 50; PABA, 15
Stress Formula w/Iron (Vita-Fresh)	x	x	30	600	400	15	15	100	25	12	x	20	Fe, 27
Stress Formula Vitalizer (Taylor)	3,333	133	33	200	133	16.7	16.7	50	16.7	33.3	100	50	Ca, 200; P, 94; Cu, .67; I, .075; Fe, 9; Mg, 66.7; Zn, 5; Mn, 2.3; Cho., 33.3; inos., 33.3; PABA, 16.7; biot., 5; leci, 26.7
Stress Supplement (Plus)	x	x	x	250	50	5	5	50	5	12.5	12.5	50	Cho., 50; inos., 50; PABA, 15
Stresscaps (Lederle)	x	x	x	300	x	10	10	100	2	6	x	20	x
Stresstabs 600 (Lederle)	x	x	30	600	x	15	15	100	5	12	x	20	x

For footnotes, see page 302.

A Selected List of Multivitamin Supplements (continued)

Product (Manufacturer)	Vita-min A (IU)	Vita-min D (IU)	Vita-min E (IU)	Vita-min C (mg)	Folic Acid — (mcg)	Vita-min B₁ (mg)	Vita-min B₂ (mg)	Vita-min B₃ (mg)	Vita-min B₆ (mg)	Vita-min B₁₂ (mcg)	Bio-tin — (mcg)	Panto-thenic Acid — (mg)	Minerals & Other Nutrients[a] (mg unless noted)
Stresstabs 600 with Iron (Lederle)	x	x	30	600	400	15	15	100	25	12	x	20	Fe, 27
Stuart Formula (Stuart)	5,000	400	15	60	400	1.5	1.7	20	2	6	x	x	Ca, 160; P, 125; I, .15; Fe, 18; Mg, 100
Stuart Formula Liquid[d] (Stuart)	3,333	333	.1	x	x	1.3	1.3	10	.07	x	x	1.43	Fe, 5; Mn, .33
Stuart Hema-tinic (Stuart)	x	x	x	25	x	1.7	1.7	25	.34	2	x	1.7	Fe, 22
Stuart Hematinic Liquid[d] (Stuart)	x	x	x	x	x	1.7	1.7	10	.5	x	x	1.43	Fe, 22; Liver, 54
Stuart Prenatal (Stuart)	8,000	400	30	60	800	1.7	2	20	4	8	x	x	Ca, 200; I, .15; Fe, 60; Mg, 100
Stuart Thera-peutic (Stuart)	10,000	400	x	200	x	10	10	100	5	5	x	20	x

	A	D	E	C	FA	B₁	B₂	B₃	B₆	B₁₂	Bio	PA	Minerals/Other
Super Acu-i-tane (Alacer)	x	x	x	x	500	.75	.85	10	1	3	15	5	Selenium, 2; Chromium, 2; Amino acids, 135
Super B Complex (Nature-Made)	x	x	x	150	x	100	20	25	2	15	5	6	Liver, 100; yeast, 100
Super B Complex (Origin)	x	x	x	x	400	50	50	50	50	50	50	50	Cho., 50; inos., 10; PABA, 50
Super B Complex and C (Schiff)	x	x	x	125	50	25	25	50	25	25	25	100	Cho., 100; inos., 100; PABA, 15
Super B-Complex plus C (Radiance)	x	x	x	60	200	5	5	50	5	12.5	x	10	Cho., 25; inos., 5; PABA, 15
Super B-Complex PRN (Am. Dietaids)	x	x	x	x	400	100	100	100	100	100	100	100	Cho., 100; inos., 100; PABA, 100
Super D Cod Liver Oil₈ (Upjohn)	4,000	400	x	x	x	x	x	x	x	x	x	x	x

For footnotes, see page 302.

A Selected List of Multivitamin Supplements (continued)

Product (Manufacturer)	Vitamin A (IU)	Vitamin D (IU)	Vitamin E (IU)	Vitamin C (mg)	Folic Acid (mcg)	Vitamin B₁ (mg)	Vitamin B₂ (mg)	Vitamin B₃ (mg)	Vitamin B₆ (mg)	Vitamin B₁₂ (mcg)	Biotin (mcg)	Pantothenic Acid (mg)	Minerals & Other Nutrients[a] (mg unless noted)
Super D Perles (Upjohn)	10,000	400	x	x	x	x	x	x	x	x	x	x	x
Super Dry Vits. A & D (GNC/Nat. Sales)	10,000	400	x	x	x	x	x	x	x	x	x	x	x
Super Hi B Complex (RichLife)	x	x	x	x	50	50	12.5	75	12.5	12.5	25	12.5	Cho., 50; inos., 50; PABA, 15; liver, 50; yeast, 50
Super One Daily (RichLife)	10,000	400	50	150	100	25	25	100	25	100	20	50	Ca, 29; P, 22; Cu, 25; I, .1; Fe, 5.7; Mg, 8; Zn, .18; Mn, 6.1; Selenium, .025; Cho., 250; inos., 250; PABA, 25; biof., 55; betaine, 25; glut. acid, 25
Super Plenamins (Rexall)	8,000	400	1.8	56	x	2.3	2.35	18	1	1.5	x	x	x

	A	D	E	C	FA	B_1	B_2	B_3	B_6	B_{12}	Bio	PA	Minerals/Other
Super Plenamins with Minerals (Rexall)	8,000	400	1	75	x	2.5	2.5	20	1	3	20	3	Ca, 75; P, 58; Cu, .75; I, .15; Fe, 30; Mg, 10; Zn, 1; Mn, 1.25; Liver, 100
Super Thera-B (Stur-Dee)	x	x	x	x	133	3.3	5	8.3	3.3	8.3	33	33	Cho., 83.3; inos., 41.7; PABA, 16.7
Super-Vim 75 (Gabriel's)	10,000	400	150	250	400	75	75	75	75	75	75	75	Ca, 10; Cu, .03; I, .15; Fe, 1; Mg, 1.54; Zn, 1.5; K, 1; Mn, .61; Cho., 75; inos., 75; PABA, 75; biot., 55; betaine, 25; glut. acid, 25
Super-Yeast (Stur-Dee)	x	x	x	x	x	3	3	1	.02	10	.5	.05	P, 6; Mg, 1.8; K, 7; Cho., 1.5; inos., .2
Supreme-50 Super-B-Complex (Gabriel's)	x	x	x	x	100	50	50	50	50	50	50	50	Cho., 50; inos., 50; PABA, 50
Surbex (Abbott)	x	x	x	x	x	6	6	30	2.5	5	x	10	x
Surbex-T (Abbott)	x	x	x	500	x	15	10	100	5	10	x	20	x

For footnotes, see page 302.

287

A Selected List of Multivitamin Supplements (continued)

Product (Manufacturer)	Vitamin A (IU)	Vitamin D (IU)	Vitamin E (IU)	Vitamin C (mg)	Folic Acid (mcg)	Vitamin B$_1$ (mg)	Vitamin B$_2$ (mg)	Vitamin B$_3$ (mg)	Vitamin B$_6$ (mg)	Vitamin B$_{12}$ (mcg)	Biotin (mcg)	Pantothenic Acid (mg)	Minerals & Other Nutrients[a] (mg unless noted)
Surbex with C (Abbott)	x	x	x	250	x	6	6	30	2.5	5	x	10	x
Sustained Release B-Complex (Naturade)	x	x	x	x	400	45	51	300	60	90	50	150	Selenium, 25; Cho., 40; inos., 40
Taka-Combex (Parke-Davis)	x	x	x	30	x	10	10	10	.5	1	x	6	Liver, 340; enzymes, 162.5
Thera-Combex (Parke-Davis)	x	x	x	250	x	25	15	100	1	5	x	20	Enzymes, 162.5
Thera-Combex H-P (Parke-Davis)	x	x	x	500	x	25	15	100	10	5	x	20	x
Theragran (Squibb)	10,000	400	15	200	x	10	10	100	5	5	x	20	x

	A	D	E	C	FA	B₁	B₂	B₃	B₆	B₁₂	Bio	PA	Minerals/Other
Theragran Liquid (Squibb)	10,000	400	x	200	x	10	10	100	5	5	x	20	x
Theragran-M (Squibb)	10,000	400	15	200	x	10	10	100	5	5	x	20	Cu, 2; I, .15; Fe, 12; Mg, 65; Zn, 1.5; Mn, 1
Therapeutic Vitamins and Minerals (Nion)	10,000	400	15	200	x	10	10	100	5	5	x	20	Cu, 2; I, .15; Fe, 12; Mg, 65; Zn, 1.5; Mn, 1
Theravim (Hudson)	10,000	400	50	300	x	15	15	10	5	10	10	20	Ca, 23; P, 18; Cu, 2; Fe, 15; Mg, 65; Zn, 1.5; K, 5; Mn, 1; PABA, 10; biof., 10
Theron (Stuart)	10,000	400	x	300	x	15	10	100	5	5	x	20	Ca, 100; Fe, 15; Zn, 1.5; Mn, 1
Therovite-M (Natural Sales)	10,000	400	100	250	x	25	15	25	10	15	25	25	Ca, 125; P, 57; Cu, 2; I, .15; Fe, 15; Mg, 40; Zn, 5; Mn, 2
Thex Forte (Ingram)	x	x	x	500	x	25	15	100	5	x	x	10	x

For footnotes, see page 302.

A Selected List of Multivitamin Supplements (continued)

Product (Manufacturer)	Vitamin A (IU)	Vitamin D (IU)	Vitamin E (IU)	Vitamin C (mg)	Folic Acid — (mcg)	Vitamin B₁ (mg)	Vitamin B₂ (mg)	Vitamin B₃ (mg)	Vitamin B₆ (mg)	Vitamin B₁₂ (mcg)	Biotin — (mcg)	Pantothenic Acid — (mg)	Minerals & Other Nutrients* (mg unless noted)
Time Release B-100 (Nature's Bounty)	x	x	x	x	100	100	100	100	100	100	100	100	Cho., 100; inos, 100; PABA, 100
Timed Release B-Complex 130 (Radiance)	x	x	x	x	400	130	130	130	130	130	130	130	Cho., 130; inos, 130; PABA, 130
Tonebec (A.V.P.)	x	x	x	300	x	15	10	5	5	x	x	10	x
Toplex 500— B-Complex (Hudson)	x	x	x	500	x	25	12.5	100	10	5	x	20	x
Total-B (Natural Sales)	x	x	x	x	200	5	7.5	12.5	5	12.5	50	50	Cho., 125; inos, 125; PABA, 25
Triple-B (Biorganic)	x	x	x	x	400	10	15	25	10	25	100	100	Cho., 250; inos, 125; PABA, 50

	A	D	E	C	FA	B$_1$	B$_2$	B$_3$	B$_6$	B$_{12}$	Bio	PA	Minerals/Other
Trisorbin Drops[d] (Reid-Provident)	3,000	400	x	x	60	x	x	x	1	x	x	x	x
Tri-Vi-Sol Chewable (Mead Johnson)	2,500	400	x	x	60	x	x	x	x	x	x	x	x
Tri-Vi-Sol Drops[d] (Mead Johnson)	1,500	400	x	x	35	x	x	x	x	x	x	x	x
Tri-Vi-Sol with Iron Drops[d] (Mead Johnson)	1,500	400	x	x	35	x	x	x	x	x	x	x	Fe, 10
Troph-Iron (Smith Kline & French)	x	x	x	x	x	10	x	x	x	25	x	x	Fe, 30
Troph-Iron Liquid[d] (Smith Kline & French)	x	x	x	x	x	10	x	x	x	25	x	x	Fe, 30
Trophite (Smith Kline & French)	x	x	x	x	x	10	x	x	x	25	x	x	x

For footnotes, see page 302.

A Selected List of Multivitamin Supplements (continued)

Product (Manufacturer)	Vitamin A (IU)	Vitamin D (IU)	Vitamin E (IU)	Vitamin C (mg)	Folic Acid (mcg)	Vitamin B1 (mg)	Vitamin B2 (mg)	Vitamin B3 (mg)	Vitamin B6 (mg)	Vitamin B12 (mcg)	Biotin (mcg)	Pantothenic Acid (mg)	Minerals & Other Nutrients[a] (mg unless noted)
Tru-Vite (Schiff)	10,000	400	10	75	1.75	1.5	3	4	.02	5	.5	.04	Cho, 1.9; inos., 1.9; PABA, .003; biof., 15
Ulticaps-M (Vitamin Quota)	10,000	400	15	200	x	10	10	100	5	5	x	20	Cu, 2; I, .15; Fe, 12; Mg, 65; Zn, 1.5; Mn, 1
Ultims (Vitamin Quota)	10,000	400	50	300	x	15	10	100	5	10	10	20	Ca, 23; P, 18; Cu, 2; Fe, 15; Mg, .65; Zn, 1.5; K, 3; Mn, 1; PABA, 10; biof., 10
Ulvical Prenatal (Ulmer)	4,000	200	15	30	400	.85	1	10	1.3	4	x	x	Ca, 200; I, .075; Fe, 30; Mg, 225
Unicap (Upjohn)	5,000	400	5	45	x	2.8	3.2	36	x	x	x	x	x
Unicap Chewable (Upjohn)	4,000	400	x	75	x	2	2	18	1	2	x	5	x
Unicap Senior (Upjohn)	5,000	400	10	90	x	3	3	30	1.5	3	x	9	Ca, 50; Cu, 1; I, .15; Fe, 10; Mg, 6; K, 5; Mn, 1

292

	A	D	E	C	FA	B_1	B_2	B_3	B_6	B_{12}	Bio	PA	Minerals/Other
Unicap Therapeutic (Upjohn)	5,000	400	30	300	x	10	10	100	2	4	x	20	Ca, 50; Cu, 1; I, .15; Fe, 10; Mg, 6; K, 5; Mn, 1
V-Complette (Schiff)	3,333	133	8.3	33	.92	1	2	.67	.01	4.17	.22	.02	Ca, 125; P, 60; I, .04; Fe, 6.7; Mg, .83; Fluorine, .25; traces: Zn, Mn, Silicon; Cho., .56; inos., .7; PABA, .001; biot., 10; enzymes, 45
Vegetarian One-A-Day (RichLife)	25,000	1,000	100	300	400	25	25	25	25	25	25	25	Ca, 80; P, 62; Cu, 2; I, .1; Fe, 13.5; Mg, 40; Zn, 4; Selenium, .025; PABA, 25
Vi-Aqua (USV)	5,000	400	1	50	x	5	5	20	.5	1	x	5	x
Vi-Aqua Therapeutic (USV)	10,000	400	5	150	x	10	5	100	1	2	x	10	x
Vi-Aquamin (USV)	6,000	440	1.05	65	x	4.5	3.15	26.25	.53	1.5	x	16	Ca, 143; P, 111; Cu, 1.5; I, .1; Fe, 30; Mg, 1; Zn, 1; Mn, 1
Vi-Aquamin Therapeutic (USV)	10,000	440	5.25	150	x	15	5.25	105	1.05	7.5	x	10	Ca, 58; P, 45; Cu, 1.5; I, .1; Fe, 30; Mg, 6; Zn, 1; Mn, 1
Vicon-C (Meyer)	x	x	x	300	x	20	10	100	5	x	x	20	Mg, 70; Zn, 80

For footnotes, see page 302.

A Selected List of Multivitamin Supplements (continued)

Product (Manufacturer)	Vitamin A (IU)	Vitamin D (IU)	Vitamin E (IU)	Vitamin C (mg)	Folic Acid (mcg)	Vitamin B₁ (mg)	Vitamin B₂ (mg)	Vitamin B₃ (mg)	Vitamin B₆ (mg)	Vitamin B₁₂ (mcg)	Biotin (mcg)	Pantothenic Acid (mg)	Minerals & Other Nutrients[a] (mg unless noted)
Vicon Chewable (Meyer)	2,000	x	25	75	x	5	2.5	12.5	1	x	x	5	Mg, 35; Zn, 10; Mn, 2
Vicon Plus (Meyer)	4,000	x	50	150	x	10	5	25	2	x	x	10	Mg, 70; Zn, 80; Mn, 4
Vi-Daylin ADC Drops[e] (Ross)	1,500	400	x	60	x	x	x	x	x	x	x	x	x
Vi-Daylin Chewable (Ross)	2,500	400	10	40	200	.7	.8	9	.7	3	x	x	Sugar
Vi-Daylin Drops[e] (Ross)	1,500	400	5	35	x	.5	.6	8	.4	1.5	x	x	x
Vi-Daylin Liquid[d] (Ross)	2,500	400	15	60	x	1.05	1.2	13.5	1.05	4.5	x	x	Sugar
Vi-Daylin Over 4 Chewable (Ross)	5,000	400	30	60	400	1.5	1.7	20	2	6	x	x	Sugar

294

	A	D	E	C	FA	B_1	B_2	B_3	B_6	B_{12}	Bio	PA	Minerals/Other
Vigran (Squibb)	5,000	400	30	60	400	1.5	1.7	20	2	6	x	x	x
Vigran Chewable (Squibb)	2,500	400	10	40	200	.7	.8	9	.7	3	x	x	x
Vigran plus Iron (Squibb)	5,000	400	30	60	400	1.5	1.7	20	2	6	x	x	Fe, 27
Vim Caps 100 (Synergy Plus)	12,500	500	75	125	200	50	50	50	50	50	50	50	Ca, 25; I, .08; Fe, 5; Mg, 3.6; Zn, 7.5; K, 5; Mn, 3; traces: Selenium, Chromium; Cho., 50; inos., 50; PABA, 50; biof., 27.5; betaine, 12.5; glut., 12.5
V.I.M. for Men (Hudson)	5,000	x	15	45	400	1.4	1.6	18	x	3	x	x	Ca, 100; P, 100; I, .013; Fe, 10; Mg, 87.5; Zn, 15
V.I.M. for Women (Hudson)	4,000	x	12	45	400	1	1.2	13	2	3	x	x	Ca, 100; I, .01; Fe, 18; Mg, 75; Zn, 15
Vi-Magna (Lederle)	5,000	400	15	60	400	1.5	1.7	20	2	6	x	x	x
Vio-Bec (Rowell)	x	x	x	500	x	25	25	100	25	x	x	40	x

For footnotes, see page 302.

A Selected List of Multivitamin Supplements (continued)

Product (Manufacturer)	Vitamin A (IU)	Vitamin D (IU)	Vitamin E (IU)	Vitamin C (mg)	Folic Acid (mcg)	Vitamin B1 (mg)	Vitamin B2 (mg)	Vitamin B3 (mg)	Vitamin B6 (mg)	Vitamin B12 (mcg)	Biotin (mcg)	Pantothenic Acid (mg)	Minerals & Other Nutrients[a] (mg unless noted)
Vio-Geric (Rowell)	5,000	400	30	60	400	5	5	20	2.4	6	x	x	Ca, 220; P, 125; Cu, 2; I, .15; Fe, 18; Mg, 100; Zn, 15
Vi-Penta Infant Drops[b] (Roche)	5,000	400	2	50	x	x	x	x	x	x	x	x	x
Vi-Penta Multivitamin Drops[b] (Roche)	5,000	400	2	50	x	1	1	10	1	x	30	11.6	x
Viri-lets (Owen)	x	x	100	50	x	5	5	50	12.5	5	x	10	x
Vi-Syneral Basic Vitamin Drops[b] (Fisons)	5,000	400	5	60	x	x	x	x	x	x	x	x	x
Vi-Syneral One-Caps (Fisons)	5,000	x	30	60	400	1.5	1.7	20	2	6	x	x	Fe, 18
Vita-Cal (Shaklee)	x	66.7	x	x	x	1	1	x	x	x	x	x	Ca, 750; P, 500

	A	D	E	C	FA	B₁	B₂	B₃	B₆	B₁₂	Bio	PA	Minerals/Other
Vita-Kaps (Abbott)	5,000	400	x	50	x	3	2.5	20	.5	2	x	5	x
Vita-Kaps-M (Abbott)	5,000	400	x	50	x	3	2.5	20	.5	2	x	5	Cu, 1; I, .15; Fe, 10; Mg, 5; Zn, 1.5; Mn, 1
Vital-B for Men (Centre City Corp.)	x	x	100	x	x	25	x	x	50	100	x	x	Zn, 15; Mn, 5
Vital-B for Women (Centre City Corp.)	x	x	100	x	x	25	x	x	50	100	x	x	Fe, 18; Zn, 15; Mn, 5
Vitamin and Mineral Supplement (Caps. or Tabs.) (Plus)	10,000	400	20	100	100	5	5	40	5	10	25	20	Ca, 102; P, 46; Cu, .5; I, 1; Fe, 15; Mg, 48; Zn, 1; K, 10; Mn, 1; Cho., 31.4; inos., 25; PABA, 30; biof., 35; lysine, 20
Vitamin B Complex (McKesson)	x	x	x	x	x	1.5	2	10	.25	.5	x	.5	Brewers yeast, 275
Vitamin B Complex—Basic Formula (Taylor)	x	x	x	x	200	5	5	50	5	37.5	150	25	Cho., 10; inos., 10; PABA, 15; yeast, .25

For footnotes, see page 302.

A Selected List of Multivitamin Supplements (continued)

Product (Manufacturer)	Vitamin A (IU)	Vitamin D (IU)	Vitamin E (IU)	Vitamin C (mg)	Folic Acid (mcg)	Vitamin B₁ (mg)	Vitamin B₂ (mg)	Vitamin B₃ (mg)	Vitamin B₆ (mg)	Vitamin B₁₂ (mcg)	Biotin (mcg)	Pantothenic Acid (mg)	Minerals & Other Nutrients[a] (mg unless noted)
Vitamin B Complex Elixir (Parke-Davis)	x	x	x	x	x	1.5	.8	10	1	x	x	5	Alcohol, 15%
Vitamin B Complex 125 SR (Taylor)	x	x	x	x	400	125	125	125	125	125	125	125	Cho, 125; inos, 125; PABA, 125
Vitamin B Complex Syrup with Iron (Plus)	x	x	x	x	100	5	5	30	5	10	15	50	Fe, 20; Cho, 60; inos, 60; PABA, 30
Vitamin B Complex w/C (McKesson)	x	x	x	300	x	15	10	50	5	x	x	10	x
Vitamin B-Complex w/Chol. & Inos. (Basic Organics)	x	x	x	x	16.7	.8	.8	8.3	.8	4.2	4.2	3.3	Cho,. 166.7; inos, 166.7; PABA, 6.7

	A	D	E	C	FA	B$_1$	B$_2$	B$_3$	B$_6$	B$_{12}$	Bio	PA	Minerals/Other
Vitamin Syrup[d] (Plus)	10,000	400	5	50	x	2	2	10	2	5	30	20	x
Vitamins A & D (RichLife)	10,000	400	x	x	x	x	x	x	x	x	x	x	x
Vitamins A & D Drops[j] (Schiff)	5,000	400	x	x	x	x	x	x	x	x	x	x	x
Vitamins A & D Perles (Plus)	10,000	400	x	x	x	x	x	x	x	x	x	x	x
Vitamins A & D Tablets (Plus)	10,000	400	x	x	x	x	x	x	x	x	x	x	x
Vitamins A, D & E (Plus)	10,000	400	300	x	x	x	x	x	x	x	x	x	x
Vitamins A, D, E, & F (NuLife)	10,000	200	200	x	x	x	x	x	x	x	x	x	Leci., 100
Vitamins C & E Chewable (Hudson)	x	x	400	500	x	x	x	x	x	x	x	x	x

For footnotes, see page 302.

A Selected List of Multivitamin Supplements (continued)

Product (Manufacturer)	Vitamin A (IU)	Vitamin D (IU)	Vitamin E (IU)	Vitamin C (mg)	Folic Acid — (mcg)	Vitamin B_1 (mg)	Vitamin B_2 (mg)	Vitamin B_3 (mg)	Vitamin B_6 (mg)	Vitamin B_{12} (mcg)	Biotin — (mcg)	Pantothenic Acid — (mg)	Minerals & Other Nutrients[a] (mg unless noted)
Vitamins C and E 1000 (Parke-Davis)	x	x	500	500	x	x	x	x	x	x	x	x	x
Vitaplex (Thompson)	10,000	400	100	250	400	30	30	100	30	250	15	100	Ca, 30; P, 15; Fe, 18; Mg, 20; Zn, 5; K, 2; Mn, 7; Cho, 50; inos, 50; PABA, 30; biof, 55; betaine, 5
Viterra High Potency (Pfipharmecs)	10,000	400	5	150	x	10.3	10	100.8	1.65	5	x	4.6	Ca, 50; Cu, 1; I, .15; Fe, 10; Mg, 5; Zn, 1.2; Mn, 1
Viterra 100% RDA (Pfipharmecs)	5,000	400	30	60	400	1.5	1.7	20	2	6	x	x	x
Viterra Original Formulation (Pfipharmecs)	5,000	400	3.7	50	x	3.09	3	25.2	.82	2	x	4.6	Ca, 110; P, 40; Cu, 1; I, .15; Fe, 10; Mg, 5; Zn, 1.2; Mn, 1
Vi-True (Schiff)	5,000	400	10	50	x	1.5	1.5	5	x	10	x	x	Biof., 12.5

	A	D	E	C	FA	B_1	B_2	B_3	B_6	B_{12}	Bio	PA	Minerals/Other
Vi-Zac (Meyer)	5,000	x	50	500	x	x	x	x	x	x	x	x	Zn, 80
Wheat Germ Oil (Schiff)	2,500	37.5	x	x	x	x	x	x	x	x	x	x	x
Yeast 500 Powder (Westpro)	x	x	x	x	100	8	8	40	8	12	25	32	Ca, 375; P, 375; Cu, .28; I, .1; Fe, 5; Mg, 150; Zn, 2; K, 320; Mn, 56; Sodium, 32; Cho, 88; inos, 64; PABA, 30
Yeast Tablets (Squibb)	x	x	x	x	x	.68	.34	2	x	x	x	x	Protein, 2% RDA
Youngstar (Schiff)	1,500	100	1.25	30	x	.37	.75	.13	x	2.5	x	x	Ca, 37.5; I, .03; Fe, 3.75; Biof., 12.5; lysine, 12.5
Zacne (Nature's Bounty)	500	x	25	75	x	x	x	x	10	x	x	x	Zn, 25
Z-Bec (Robins)	x	x	45	600	x	15	10.2	100	10	6	x	25	Zn, 22.5
Zentinic (Lilly)	x	x	x	200	50	7.5	7.5	30	7.5	50	x	15	Fe, 100
Zentron[d] (Lilly)	x	x	x	100	x	1	1	5	1	5	x	1	Fe, 20

For footnotes, see page 302.

A Selected List of Multivitamin Supplements (continued)

Product (Manufacturer)	Vitamin A (IU)	Vitamin D (IU)	Vitamin E (IU)	Vitamin C (mg)	Folic Acid – (mcg)	Vitamin B1 (mg)	Vitamin B2 (mg)	Vitamin B3 (mg)	Vitamin B6 (mg)	Vitamin B12 (mcg)	Biotin – (mcg)	Pantothenic Acid – (mg)	Minerals & Other Nutrients[a] (mg unless noted)
Zymacap (Upjohn)	5,000	400	x	100	x	5	5	30	2	4	x	10	x
Zymadrops[b] (Upjohn)	2,000	400	x	50	x	1	1	10	1	x	x	3	x
Zymalixir Syrup[d] (Upjohn)	x	x	x	x	x	1	1	8	.5	2	x	x	Fe, 15; Liver, 65
Zymasyrup[d] (Upjohn)	5,000	400	x	60	x	1	1	10	.5	3	x	3	x
Zymatinic Drops[b] (Upjohn)	x	x	x	x	x	.6	.6	4.8	.3	.6	x	x	Liver, 39

a. Cho. = choline; inos. = inositol; PABA = para aminobenzoic acid; biof. = bioflavonoids, including rutin, hesperidin; leci. = lecithin; *amino acids:* betaine, glut. = glutamic acid, lysine, meth. = methionine; *antihistamine:* phenylpropanolamine; *nucleic acid:* RNA, others; *detergent:* DDS = dioctyl sodium sulfosuccinate; *liver:* delivered in various forms (dry, desiccated, fractions, whole, defatted).
b. Per 6 ml.
c. Per tablespoon (15 ml).
d. Per teaspoon (5 ml).
e. Per 4 tablespoons (60 ml).
f. Per 2 tablespoons (30 ml or 1 fluid ounce).
g. Per ml.
h. Per 1/3 teaspoon.
i. Per .2 ml.

A Selected List of Single Vitamin Supplements

Key: *Units:* IU = international units; mg = milligrams; mcg = micrograms.
Vitamins: Vitamin D (calciferol, cholecalciferol, or ergocalciferol); Vitamin E (tocopherol); Vitamin C (ascorbic acid or sodium ascorbate); Folic Acid (folate or folacin);
Vitamin B_1 (thiamin or thiamine); Vitamin B_2 (riboflavin); Vitamin B_3 (niacin, niacinamide, nicotinic acid, or nicotinamide); Vitamin B_6 (pyridoxine); Vitamin B_{12} (cobalamin
or cyanocobalamin); Pantothenic Acid (panthenol, calcium pantothenate, calcium pantothenate, pantothenyl alcohol, or dexpanthenol).
Minerals: Ca (calcium); P (phosphorus); Cu (Copper); I (iodine); Fe (iron); Mg (magnesium); Zn (zinc); K (potassium); Mn (manganese).

VITAMIN A

Product (Manufacturer)	IU	Minerals & Other Nutrients[a] (mg unless noted)
Alphalin (Lilly)	10,000	x
Aquasol A Capsules (USV)	27,500 55,000	x
Carrot Oil Capsules (Biorganic)	10,000	x
Emulsified A (Schiff)	10,000	x
Golden Bounty Vitamin A (Squibb)	10,000	x

Vitamin A cont'd

Product (Manufacturer)	IU	Minerals & Other Nutrients[a] (mg unless noted)
Lecithal (Schiff)	1,000	Phosphatide, 370
Natural Vitamin A (Basic Organics)	25,000	x
Sust-A-5 (Miller)	5,000	x
Vitamin A (GNC/Nat. Sales)	10,000 25,000	x x
Vitamin A (McKesson)	10,000	x
Vitamin A (Plus)	10,000	x
Vitamin A (RichLife)	10,000 25,000	x x

303

Vitamin A cont'd		
Product (Manufacturer)	IU	Minerals & Other Nutrients[a] (mg unless noted)
Vitamin A (Schein)	10,000 25,000 50,000	x
Vitamin A (Schiff)	10,000	x
Vitamin A (Squibb)	10,000	x
Vitamin A (Sundown)	10,000	x
Vitamin A, Dry (RichLife)	10,000	x
Vitamin A, Emulsified (Plus)	10,000	x

Vitamin D cont'd		
Product (Manufacturer)	IU	Minerals & Other Nutrients[a] (mg unless noted)
Vitamin D (GNC/ Nat. Sales)	400 1,000	x
Vitamin D (RichLife)	400 1,000	x

VITAMIN E		
Product (Manufacturer)	IU	Minerals & Other Nutrients[a] (mg unless noted)
Aquasol E (USV)	30 100 400	x
Dry All-E (Schiff)	100 200 400	x
E 1000 (F&F)	71	x
E-Chew (Schiff)	100 200	x

VITAMIN D

Product (Manufacturer)	IU	Minerals & Other Nutrients[a] (mg unless noted)
Bone Meal Tablets (RichLife)	100	Ca, 214.5; P, 97.5
Calcicaps (Nion)	67	Ca, 125; P, 60
Calcicaps with Iron (Nion)	67	Ca, 125; P, 60; Fe, 13
Calcium Malties Chewable Wafers (RichLife)	80	Ca, 200; P, 150; Mg, 12.5
Chew-Mins (Schiff)	80	Ca, 200; P, 100; Mg, 12.5
Dical-D Caps. (Abbott)	133	Ca, 117; P, 90
Dical-D Wafers (Abbott)	200	Ca, 232; P, 180
Dical-D with Iron (Abbott)	133	Ca, 147; P, 114; Fe, 10
Os-Cal (Marion)	125	Ca, 250

Vitamin E cont'd

Product (Manufacturer)	IU	Pectin, 100 200
Emulsified Vitamin E (Plus)	100, 200	x
Eprolin (Lilly)	50, 100	
Golden Bounty Vitamin E (Squibb)	100, 200, 400	x
Natural Vitamin E (Alpha Tocopherol, Caps.) (Plus)	100, 200, 300, 400, 500, 600, 800	x
Natural Vitamin E (Alpha Tocopherol, Caps.) (RichLife)	100, 200, 400, 1,000	x
NF&V Natural Vitamin E (McKesson)	100, 200, 400	x

Vitamin E cont'd

Product (Manufacturer)	IU	Minerals & Other Nutrients[a] (mg unless noted)
Pheryl-E (Miller)	100 400	x
Super Golden E (Westpro)	200	Leci, 300; wheat germ oil, 300
Vitamin E (Am. Dietaids)	1,000	x
Vitamin E (Hudson)	100 200 400 600 1,000	x
Vitamin E (McKesson)	100 200 400	x
Vitamin E (Squibb)	100	x

VITAMIN C

Product (Manufacturer)	mg	Minerals & Other Nutrients[a] (mg unless noted)
Acerola Chews (Plus)	100	x
Acerola Plus (Am. Dietaids)	100	Biof, 25
Ascorbic Acid Coated Tabs. (Person & Covey)	500	x
Bio-Gram (Alacer)	100	Biof, 1,000
Buffered C (Thompson)	500 1,000	x
Buffered Summa C (Radiance)	1,500	Rose hips, 150
"C" Bioflavonoids (Solgar)	100	Biof, 125

Vitamin 'E' cont'd

Vitamin E (Wampole)	100 200 400 800	x
Vitamin E Dry (Solgar)	400	x
Vitamin E Natural (Parke-Davis)	200 400	x
Vitamin E Synthetic (Parke-Davis)	200 400	x
Vitamin E Walnut-Flavored Tablets (Squibb)	200 400	x
Water Dispersible Nat. E-400 (Naturade)	400	x
Wheat Germ Olic (Plus)	30	x
Wheat Germ Oil Perles (Plus)	1.8	x

Vitamin C cont'd

C + Rose Hips (Schiff)	250 500 1,000		x
C Speridin (Marlyn)	200	Biof., 200	
Cal-Ascorbs (Alacer)	450	Ca, 50	
Cemill (Miller)	250 500		x
Cevalin (Lilly)	50 100 250 500		x
Cevi-Bid (Geriatric)	500		x
Ce-Vi-Sol Drops* (Mead Johnson)	35	Alcohol, 5%	
Chewable Orange C-500 (Thompson)	500		x

Vitamin C cont'd

Product (Manufacturer)	mg	Minerals & Other Nutrients[a] (mg unless noted)
Chewable Vitamin C (McKesson)	100 250	x
Chewable Vit. C (Wampole)	100 250 500	x
Controlled Release C-1000 (Thompson)	1,000	x
C-Ron (Rowell)	100	Fe, 66
C-Ron Forte (Rowell)	600	Fe, 66
C-Ron Freckles (Rowell)	50	Fe, 33
C-Vi-Complex (Schiff)	500	Biof., 150
Daily C (F&F)	250	x

Vitamin C cont'd

Product (Manufacturer)	mg	Minerals & Other Nutrients[a] (mg unless noted)
Pure Ascorbic Acid (Plus)	500	x
Pure Ascorbic Acid Powder (Plus)	1,500	x
Recoup (Lederle)	300	Fe, 50; DSS, 50
Rose Hips (Solgar)	250 500	x
Rose Hips C (Plus)	500 600 1,000	x
Special C-500 (Gabriel's)	500	Biof, 176
Spider-man C (Hudson)	60	x
Super C-500 (Sundown)	500	Biof, 175

Vitamin C cont'd

	Dose	Other	
Ferancee-HP (Stuart)	600	Fe, 110	
Hi-C-Plex 500 (Barth's)	500	Biof., 175	
Hy-C (Solgar)	500	Biof., 175	
Instant C[c] (Westpro)	1,540		x
Liquid C-Rose Hips[c] (Basic Organics)	300		x
Mag-Ascorbs (Alacer)	470	Mg, 30	
NF&V Rose Hips Vitamin C (McKesson)	250 500		x
One Gram Vit. C (Naturade)	1,000	Biof., 25	
Peridin-C (Beutlich)	200	Biof., 200	

Vitamin C cont'd

	Dose	Biof.	
Sust. Release Vit. C (Naturade)	800	Biof., 200	x
Timed Rel. Vit. C w/Rose Hips (Origin)	500 1,000		x
Vitamin C (McKesson)	100 250 500		x
Vitamin C (Parke-Davis)	100 250 500		x
Vitamin C (RichLife)	250 500 1,000		x
Vitamin C (Squibb)	100 250 500		x
Vitamin C (Thompson)	500	Biof., 24	
Vitamin C (Vita-Fresh)	100 250 500 1,000		x

Vitamin C cont'd

Product (Manufacturer)	mg	Minerals & Other Nutrients[a] (mg unless noted)
Vitamin C Complex (RichLife)	350	Biof., 420
Vitamin C Crystals[c] (Radiance)	5,000	x
Vitamin C Granules[f] (RichLife)	1,250	x
Vit. C Nectar w/ Rose Hips (Radiance)	300	x
Vitamin C Sugar Free Liquid[c] (Schiff)	300	x
Vitamin C Timed Release (RichLife)	500	x
Vitamin C with Bioflavonoids (Plus)	200	Biof., 275

Folic Acid cont'd

Product (Manufacturer)	mcg	Minerals & Other Nutrients[a] (mg unless noted)
Fruit-of-the-Land Folic Acid (Sharpe)	400	x
High Potency Folic Acid (RichLife)	800	x

VITAMIN B₁

Product (Manufacturer)	mg	Minerals & Other Nutrients[a] (mg unless noted)
Betalin S (Lilly)	10 25 50 100	x
Betalin S Elixir[c] (Lilly)	2.25	Alcohol, 10%

Vitamin C cont'd

Product (Manufacturer)			Minerals & Other Nutrients[a] (mg unless noted)
Vitamin C with Rose Hips (RichLife)	250	500	1,000	x
Vitron-C (Fisons)	125	Fe, 66
Zinc-Ascorbs (Alacer)	180	Zn, 20

FOLIC ACID

Product (Manufacturer)	mcg	Minerals & Other Nutrients[a] (mg unless noted)
Folic Acid (Basic Organics)	800	x
Folic Acid (Schein)	100	x
Folic Acid (Solgar)	400	x
Folic Acid (Vitamin Quota)	400	x
Folvron (Lederle)	330	Fe, 57

Vitamin B₁ cont'd

Product (Manufacturer)		
Bewon Elixir[c] (Wyeth)	.25	x
B1 (RichLife)	100	x
Hi-B-1 (Hudson)	500	x
Thiamine Hydrochloride, USP (Parke-Davis)	50 100	x x
Vitamin B₁ (McKesson)	50 100	x x
Vitamin B1 (Plus)	100	x
Vitamin B1 (Schein)	10 25 50 100 250	x
Vitamin B-1 (Solgar)	50 500	x

VITAMIN B₂

Product (Manufacturer)	mg	Minerals & Other Nutrients[a] (mg unless noted)
B2 (RichLife)	50	x
B-2 (Thompson)	25 50 100 250	x
Riboflavin (Lilly)	5 10	x
Vitamin B-2 (GNC/ Nat. Sales)	50 100 250	x
Vitamin B2 (Plus)	10	x
Vitamin B-2 (Solgar)	25 50 100	x

Vitamin B₃ cont'd

Product (Manufacturer)	mg	Minerals & Other Nutrients[a] (mg unless noted)
Nicotinex Elixir[c] (Fleming)	50	Alcohol, 18%
Nicotinic Acid (Parke-Davis)	50 100	x
SK-Niacin (Smith Kline & French)	50 100	x

VITAMIN B₆

Product (Manufacturer)	mg	Minerals & Other Nutrients[a] (mg unless noted)
B6 (RichLife)	50 100	x
B-6 (Thompson)	25 50 100 250 500	x

312

VITAMIN B₃

Product (Manufacturer)	mg	Minerals & Other Nutrients[a] (mg unless noted)
Niacin (Lilly)	20 50 100	x
Niacin (McKesson)	50 100	x
Niacin (Plus)	100	x
Niacin (RichLife)	100	x
Niacin (Squibb)	25 50 100 500	x
Niacinamide (Lilly)	50 100	x
Niacinamide (Plus)	200	x
Niacinamide (RichLife)	100 500	x

Vitamin B₆ cont'd

Product (Manufacturer)	mg	Minerals & Other Nutrients[a] (mg unless noted)
B6 (Westpro)	500	x
Formula 50 (Marlyn)	1	Amino acids, 500
Formula TR (Westpro)	5	Ca, 25; Mg, 25; K, 99
Hi-B-6 (Hudson)	500	x
Lecithin 1200 (RichLife)	16.7	Leci., 400; kelp, 50; vinegar, 80
Nature's Wonder (Ford)	3.5	Leci, 100; kelp, 25; vinegar, 40
Vitamin B-6 (Am. Dietaids)	25	x
Vitamin B-6 (Basic Organics)	50 100 250	x
Vitamin B₆ (McKesson)	25 50	x

Vitamin B6 cont'd

Product (Manufacturer)	mg	Minerals & Other Nutrients[a] (mg unless noted)
Vitamin B6 (Plus)	10 25 50	x
Vitamin B6 (Wampole)	25 100	x

VITAMIN B12

Product (Manufacturer)	mcg	Minerals & Other Nutrients[a] (mg unless noted)
B12 (RichLife)	100 500 1,500	x
B-12 (Thompson)	50 100 250 500 1,000	x
Hi-B-12 (Hudson)	2,000	x

Vitamin B12 cont'd

Product (Manufacturer)	mcg	Minerals & Other Nutrients[a] (mg unless noted)
Vitamin B12 (Schiff)	25 100 250	x
Vitamin B12 (Squibb)	25	x
Vitamin B-12 (Vita-Fresh)	50 100 250 500	x

BIOTIN

Product (Manufacturer)	mcg	Minerals & Other Nutrients[a] (mg unless noted)
Biotin (GNC/Nat. Sales)	50 300	x
Biotin (Plus)	50	x
Biotin (RichLife)	300	x

Vitamin B-12 cont'd

Product	mg	Minerals & Other Nutrients
Nat. Vit. B-12 Lozenge (Synergy Plus)	500	x
RNA and Vitamin B12 (Westpro)	12.5	RNA, 50
Stuart Amino Acids & B12 Tabs. (Stuart)	.1	Amino acids, 600
Vitamin B-12 (Basic Organics)	50 100 250 500	x
Vitamin B-12 (GNC/Nat. Sales)	25 50 500 1,000	x
Vitamin B12 (McKesson)	25 50 100	x
Vitamin B12 (Plus)	25	x

PANTOTHENIC ACID

Product (Manufacturer)	mg	Minerals & Other Nutrients[a] (mg unless noted)
Pantothenic Acid (Plus)	100 300	x
Pantothenic Acid (Radiance)	100 250 500	x
Pantothenic Acid (RichLife)	100 250	x
Pantothenic Acid (Schein)	100	x
Timed Release Panto. Acid (Radiance)	1,000	x

CONTESTED VITAMINS

Product (Manufacturer)	Con. Vita. (mg)	Minerals & Other Nutrients[a] (mg unless noted)
Bioflavonoids (Basic Organics)	Biof., 1,000	x
Choline (Solgar)	Cho., 650	x
Choline/Inositol (Thompson)	Cho., 300, inos., 300	x
Duo-CVP (USV)	Biof., 200	x
Inositol (Plus)	Inos., 250	x
Inositol (RichLife)	Inos., 500	x
Inositol Powders (Plus)	Inos., 500	x
Lecithin Granules[h] (Emenel)	Cho., 250, inos., 250	P, 225

Contested Vitamins cont'd

Product (Manufacturer)	Con. Vita. (mg)	Minerals & Other Nutrients[a] (mg unless noted)
Lemon Biof. Complex (Radiance)	Biof., 1,000	x
Lemon Bioflavs (Alacer)	Biof., 500	x
Mega-Bio (RichLife)	Biof., 1,000	x
PABA (GNC/Nat. Sales)	PABA, 50 100 500	x
PABA (RichLife)	PABA, 100	x
Rutin (GNC/Nat. Sales)	Rutin, 20 50	x
Timed-Release PABA (Radiance)	PABA, 1,000	x

a. Cho. = choline; inos. = inositol; PABA = para aminobenzoic acid; biof. = bioflavonoids, including rutin, hesperidin, acerola; leci. = lecithin; *amino acid*: meth. = methionine, others; *detergent*: DDS = dioctyl sodium sulfosuccinate; RNA (a nucleic acid); *analgesic*: salicylamide (see Chapter 1, Robert J. Benowicz: *Non-Prescription Drugs and Their Side Effects*, N.Y.: Grosset & Dunlap, 1977); *liver*: delivered in various forms (dry, desiccated, fractions, whole, defatted).
b. Per ml.
c. Per teaspoon (5 ml).
d. Per .12-ml drop.
e. Per .6 ml.
f. Per ½ teaspoon.
g. Per ¼ teaspoon.
h. Per tablespoon.

DIRECTORY OF AMERICAN AND CANADIAN VITAMIN MANUFACTURERS

If you have questions about any vitamin supplement, it is appropriate for you to contact the manufacturer for answers. Most companies have consumer service departments that will rapidly respond to any inquiry, provide you with descriptive materials about their formulations, and send you complete product catalogues upon request.

Abbott Laboratories
North Chicago, IL
60064

Alacer Corp.
7425 Orangethorpe Ave.
Buena Park, CA
90621

American Dietaids Co., Inc.
33 Kings Hwy.
Orangeburg, NY
10962

Ayerst Laboratories
685 Third Ave.
New York, NY
10017

Barth's Nutritional Supplements
270 W. Merrick Rd.
Valley Stream, NY
11852

Basic Organics
345 N. Baldwin Park Blvd.
City of Industry, CA
91746

Beach Pharmaceuticals
5220 S. Manhattan Ave.
Tampa, FL
33611

Beecham Laboratories
501 Fifth St.
Bristol, TN 37620

Beutlich, Inc.
7006 Western Ave.
Chicago, IL
60645

Bio-Organic Brands, Inc.
26 W. Park Ave.
Long Beach, NY
11561

Bowman Pharmaceuticals
5801 Mayfair Road, N.W.
North Canton, OH
44720

Bristol-Myers Products
345 Park Ave.
New York, NY
10022

Campana Corp.
P.O. Box 6200
Carson, CA
90749

DaVinci/Sport Science
1 Executive Drive
South Burlington, VT
05401

Dista Products Co.
P.O. Box 618
Indianapolis, IN 46206

F & F Lab, Inc.
Chicago, IL
60632

Fisons Corp.
Two Preston Court
Bedford, MA
01730

Fleming & Co.
1600 Fenpark Dr.
Fenton, MO
63026

FoodScience Laboratories
1 Executive Dr.
South Burlington, VT
05401

Genovese Drug Stores, Inc.
80 Marcus Dr.
Melville, NY
11746

Geriatric Pharmaceutical Corp.
Floral Park, NY
11001

GNC (General Nutrition Corp.)
418 Wood St.
Pittsburgh, PA
15222

Hudson Pharmaceutical Corp.
21 Henderson Dr.
West Caldwell, NJ
07006

Ingram Pharmaceutical Co.
202 Green St.
San Francisco, CA
94111

Laser, Inc.
2000 N. Main St.
Crown Point, IN 46307

Lederle Laboratories
Pearl River, NY
10965

P. Leiner Nutritional Products
1845 W. 205th St.
Torrance, CA
90501

Lilly and Co., Eli
307 E. McCarty
P.O. Box 618
Indianapolis, IN 46206

Marion Laboratories, Inc.
10236 Bunker Ridge Rd.
Kansas City, MO
64137

Marlyn Pharmaceutical Co., Inc.
18261 Enterprise Lane
Huntington Beach, CA
92648

McKesson Laboratories
424 Grasmere Ave.
Fairfield, CT 06430

Mead Johnson & Co.
2404 W. Pennsylvania St.
Evansville, IN
47721

Merrell-National Laboratories
c/o Richardson-Merrell, Inc.
Cincinnati, OH
45215

Meyer Laboratories, Inc.
1900 W. Commercial Blvd.
Ft. Lauderdale, FL
33309

Miles Laboratories, Inc.
P.O. Box 340
Elkart, IN
46515

Naturite Health Products
(also Fulvita)
13260 Moore St.
Cerritos, CA 90701

Miller Pharmacal
1425 Melody Drive
Metairie, LA
70002

Nion Corp.
11581 Federal Ave.
El Monte, CA
91731

Mission Pharmacal Co.
P.O. Box 1676
San Antonio, TX
78296

North American Pharmacal, Inc.
6851 Chase Rd.
Dearborn, MI
48126

Naturade Products, Inc.
7110 E. Jackson St.
Paramount, CA
90723

NuLife, Inc.
1339 W. Gaylor
Long Beach, CA
90813

Natural Organics, Inc.
10 Daniel St.
Farmingdale, NY
11735

Parke-Davis
201 Tabor Rd.
Morris Plains, NJ
07950

Natural Sales Co.
P.O. Box 25
Pittsburgh, PA
15230

Person & Covey, Inc.
616 Allen Ave.
Glendale, CA
91201

Nature Food Centres
1 Nature's Way
Wilmington, MA 01887

Pfipharmecs
235 E. 42nd St.
New York, NY 10017

Nature-Made
(*See* Pharmavite)

Pharmavite Pharmaceutical Corp.
(Nature-Made)
12801 Rangoon St.
Pacoima, CA 91331

Nature's Bounty
105 Orville Dr.
Bohemia, NY 11716

Plus Products
2681 Kelvin Ave.
Irvine, CA 92714

Nature's Plus
10 Daniel St.
Farmingdale, NY 11735

Purex
(*See* Campana)

Radiance Products Co.
345 N. Baldwin Park Ave.
City of Industry, CA
91746

Reid-Provident Laboratories, Inc.
25 Fifth St., N.W.
Atlanta, GA
30308

Rexall Drug Co.
3901 N. Kingshighway Blvd.
St. Louis, MO
63115

Richards Laboratories, Inc.
Box 9000
Ft. Lauderdale, FL
33310

Richlife, Inc.
2211 E. Orangewood Ave.
Anaheim, CA
92806

Robins Co., A.H.
1407 Cummings Ave.
Richmond, VA
23220

Roche Laboratories
Nutley, NJ
07110

Ross Laboratories
Columbus, OH
43216

Rowell Laboratories, Inc.
210 Main St., W.
Baudette, MN
56623

RVP Vitamin Products
16 Nassau Ave.
Rockville Centre, NY
11570

Schein, Inc., Henry
39–01 170th St.
Brooklyn, NY
11358

Schering Corp.
Galloping Hill Rd.
Kenilworth, NJ
07033

Schiff Bio-Foods Products
121 Moonachie Ave.
Moonachie, NJ
07074

SDA Pharmaceuticals, Inc.
919 Third Ave.
New York, NY
10022

Shaklee Products
444 Market St.
San Francisco, CA
94111

Smith, Kline & French
1500 Spring Garden St.
P.O. Box 7929
Philadelphia, PA 19101

Smith, Miller & Patch
455 E. Middlefield Rd.
Mountain View, CA 94043

Solar Food Products
51–02 23rd
Long Island City, NY 11101

Solgar Co., Inc.
410 Ocean Ave.
Lynbrook, NY
11563

Squibb & Sons, Inc.
Lawrenceville-Princeton Rd.
Princeton, NJ
08540

S.S.S. Company
71 University Avenue, S.W.
Atlanta, GA
30315

Stuart Pharmaceuticals
Wilmington, DE
19897

Stur-Dee Health Products, Inc.
222 Livingston
Brooklyn, NY
11201

Sundown Vitamins, Inc.
Box 60–1051
North Miami Beach, FL
33160

Synergy Plus
2530 Polk St.
Union, NJ
07083

Taylor-Care
8450 Hickman Rd.
Des Moines, IA
50322

Thompson Co., Wm. T.
23529 S. Figueroa St.
Carson, CA
90745

Ulmer Pharmacal Co.
2440 Fernbrook Lane
Minneapolis, MN
55441

Upjohn Company, Inc., The
7000 Portage Rd.
Kalamazoo, MI
49001

USV Laboratories
1 Scarsdale Rd.
Tuckahoe, NY
10707

Vita-Fresh Vitamin Co.
12132 Knott St.
Garden Grove, CA 92641

Vitamerica, Inc.
760 Summer St.
Stamford, CT
06901

Vitamin Quota, Inc.
Fairfield, NJ
07006

Wampole, Inc.
180 Duncan Mill Rd.
Don Mills, Ontario, Canada
M3B 1Z6

Westpro Labs, Inc.
2211 E. Orangewood Ave.
Anaheim, CA
92806

Williams Co., Inc., The J.B.
767 Fifth Ave.
New York, NY
10022

Wyeth Laboratories
P.O. Box 8299
Philadelphia, PA
19101

An Afterword

If you have any questions about vitamins or comments about *VITAMINS & YOU,* please feel free to write to me:

Robert J. Benowicz
c/o Berkley Publishing, Inc.
200 Madison Avenue
New York, New York
10016

Although I cannot guarantee personal answers to all letters or cards, I will try—

With best wishes,

Robert J. Benowicz

ABOUT THE AUTHOR

Robert J. Benowicz is a prominent New York biochemist, author, and educator, well known for his many health-related articles in newspapers and magazines.

Selected
Bibliography

Bailey, Herbert, *Vitamin E: Your Key to a Healthy Heart* (New York: Arc Books, 1970).

Di Cyan, Erwin, Ph.D., *Vitamins in Your Life* (New York: Simon & Schuster, 1974).

Ellis, John M., M.D., and James Presley, *Vitamin B₆: The Doctor's Report* (New York: Harper & Row, 1973).

Evaluations of Drug Interactions (Washington, D.C.: American Pharmaceutical Association, 1976).

Freedland, R. A., and Stephanie Briggs, *A Biochemical Approach to Nutrition* (New York: John Wiley & Sons, 1977).

Gerras, Charles, Joseph Galant, and E. John Hanna, eds., *The Complete Book of Vitamins* (Emmaus, Pa.: Rodale Press, 1977).

Handbook of Nonprescription Drugs, fifth edition (Washington, D.C.: American Pharmaceutical Association, 1977).

Heinz Nutritional Data, sixth edition (Pittsburgh: Heinz U.S.A., 1972).

Joint FAO/WHO Expert Group, *Requirements of Ascorbic Acid, Vitamin D, Vitamin B₁₂, Folate, and Iron,* World Health Organization Technical Report Series No. 452/Food and Agriculture Organization Nutrition Meetings Report Series No. 47 (Geneva: World Health Organization, 1970).

Kutsky, Roman J., Ph.D., *Handbook of Vitamins and Hormones* (New York: Van Nostrand Reinhold, 1973).

Lehninger, Albert L., Ph.D., *Bioenergetics: The Molecular Basis of Biological Energy Transformations,* second edition (Menlo Park, Cal.: W. A. Benjamin, Inc., 1971).

Levy, Joseph V., Ph.D., and Paul Bach-y-Rita, M.D., *Vitamins: Their Use and Abuse* (New York: Liveright, 1976).

Marks, John, M.D., *A Guide to the Vitamins—Their Role in Health and Disease* (Lancaster, England: Medical & Technical Publishing).

National Research Council Food and Nutrition Board, *Recommended Dietary Allowances,* eighth and ninth editions (Washington, D.C.: National Academy of Sciences, 1974 and 1980).

Pauling, Linus, *Vitamin C, the Common Cold, and the Flu* (San Francisco: W. H. Freeman, 1976).

Physicians' Desk Reference, thirty-first edition (Oradell, N.J.: Medical Economics Co., 1977).

Roe, Daphne, M.D., *Drug-Induced Nutritional Deficiencies* (Westport, Conn.: Avi, 1976).

Rosenberg, Harold, M.D., and A. N. Feldzamen, Ph.D., *The Book of Vitamin Therapy* (New York: Berkley, 1975).

Stone, Irwin, *The Healing Factor: "Vitamin C" Against Disease* (New York: Grosset & Dunlap, 1972).

U.S. Dept. of Health, Education, and Welfare, and U.S. Food and Drug Administration, "Vitamin and Mineral Products: Labeling and Composition Regulations," in *Federal Register* (Vol. 41, Pt. V, No. 203, Oct. 19, 1976).

U.S. Senate Select Committee on Nutrition and Human Needs, *Dietary Goals for the United States* (Washington, D.C.: Government Printing Office, 1977).

INDEX

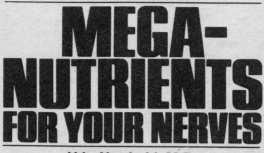